# THE COMPLETE

## CROCK POT

# Cookbook for Beginners

**1900** | Delicious & Sanity-Saving Recipes that All Ages Love to Eat, Easy Slow Cooker Cookbook from Breakfast to Desserts, Snacks, Lunch and Dinner

Kathleen J. Taylor

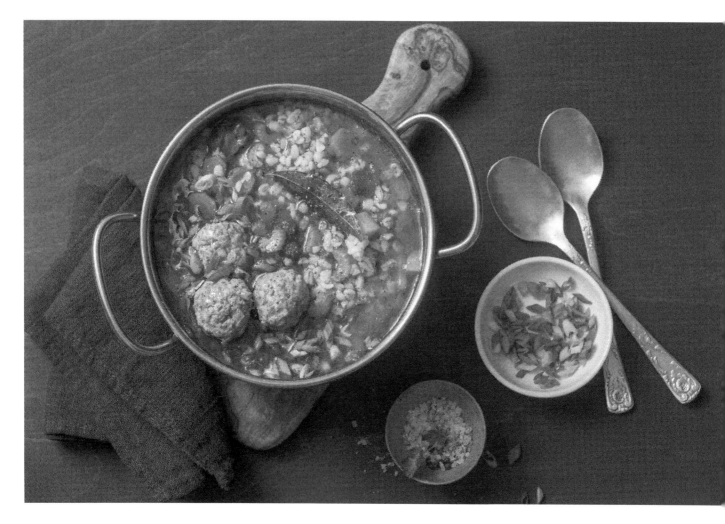

# CONTENTS

# SIDE DISH RECIPES ................................................29

# VEGETABLE & VEGETARIAN RECIPES ..................36

# LUNCH & DINNER RECIPES ..............................43

## SOUPS & STEWS RECIPES ....................................................... 50

## POULTRY RECIPES ................................................................ 57

# DESSERT RECIPES .................................................. 85

# APPENDIX A MEASUREMENT CONVERSIONS ....................... 92

# APPENDIX B : RECIPES INDEX ............................................. 94

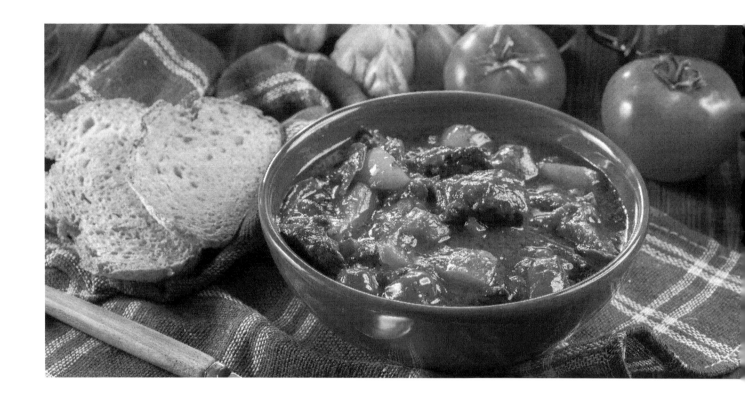

# INTRODUCTION

In the vast panorama of culinary arts, few methods conjure up the vivid tapestry of flavors, textures, and aromas quite like slow cooking. At the heart of this age-old technique is the Crock Pot, a humble kitchen appliance that has transformed countless kitchens into gourmet havens. Enter Kathleen J. Taylor—a name synonymous with culinary innovation and a fervent passion for slow-cooked delicacies.

Kathleen's journey began in the bustling heart of her grandmother's kitchen. There, surrounded by copper pots and age-old recipes, she developed an intrinsic bond with food. From the comforting embrace of hearty stews to the delicate notes of slow-cooked desserts, every meal was a lesson, every dish a treasured memory. As the years went by, Kathleen didn't just inherit a set of recipes; she was gifted a legacy—one she has since honed, expanded, and is now eager to share with the world.

This cookbook is more than just a collection of recipes. It's a testament to Kathleen's dedication to the craft, her undying love for food, and her mission to keep age-old traditions alive while infusing them with modern flair. As you turn each page, you'll discover not just the meticulous detail with which each dish has been curated but also the heart and soul that went into creating it. Kathleen's approach to slow cooking is a blend of science and art; it's about understanding the essence of each ingredient, the delicate balance of flavors, and the magic that ensues when they're brought together in the cozy cocoon of a Crock Pot.

From dishes that pay homage to her family's roots to contemporary renditions that showcase global flavors, Kathleen's cookbook is a voyage—a journey through time, cultures, and tastes. It's an exploration of the power of slow cooking to connect, to heal, and to celebrate life.

As you immerse yourself in this book, let Kathleen be your guide. Let her show you the transformative power of patience, the joy of anticipation, and the sheer delight of savoring a dish that has been lovingly crafted over hours. Welcome to "From Simmer to Sensation." Prepare to embark on an unforgettable culinary adventure.

# Benefits of Crock Pot compared to traditional cooking

Crock Pots, also known as slow cookers, offer several advantages over traditional cooking methods. Here are some of the benefits of using a Crock Pot compared to conventional cooking:

## Time-Saving

Once you prepare and add all the ingredients, the Crock Pot takes over, allowing you to set it and forget it. This frees up time for other activities or tasks without needing to constantly monitor the cooking process.

## Energy Efficiency

Slow cookers use less electricity compared to ovens or stovetops. They maintain a consistent low temperature, making them more energy-efficient over prolonged cooking durations.

## Tenderizes Meat

The long, slow cooking process helps tenderize tougher cuts of meat. As a result, less expensive cuts can be used, offering potential cost savings.

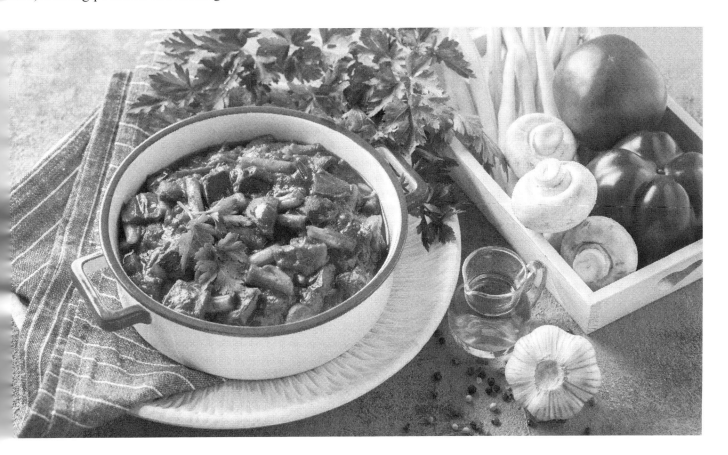

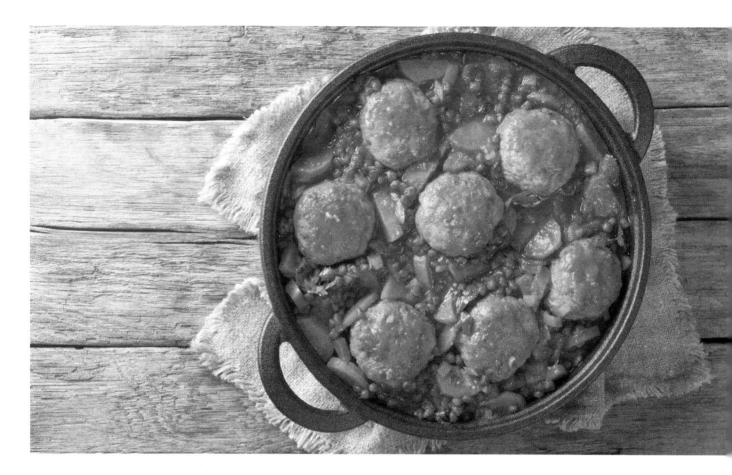

## Flavor Infusion

The extended cooking time allows flavors to meld and infuse more deeply, often resulting in richer and more flavorful dishes.

## Safety

There's a reduced risk of burning food or overcooking, and there's no open flame. For many, this offers peace of mind, especially if they're out of the house while the Crock Pot is on.

## Versatility

Crock Pots can be used to prepare a wide variety of dishes, from soups and stews to roasts, desserts, and even bread.

## One-Pot Cooking

Many Crock Pot recipes require minimal dishes or pots, reducing the cleanup time and effort.

## Consistent Results

Once you have a tried-and-true recipe, a Crock Pot provides consistent results each time, as the cooking temperature and method remain steady.

### Better Heat Distribution

The design of most Crock Pots ensures even heat distribution, preventing hot spots that can lead to uneven cooking or burnt areas.

### Maintains Moisture

The sealed or covered environment retains moisture, preventing dishes from drying out and ensuring that meats remain juicy.

In contrast, traditional cooking methods, particularly those that require continuous high heat, might require more attention and could result in uneven cooking or a loss of moisture.

## The convenience that the Crock Pot Cookbook can provide

The Crock Pot Cookbook brings a realm of convenience to both novice and seasoned cooks.

### "Set and Forget" Approach

The cookbook harnesses the Crock Pot's primary advantage – you can prepare your ingredients, set your pot, and move on with your day. No constant monitoring or stirring required.

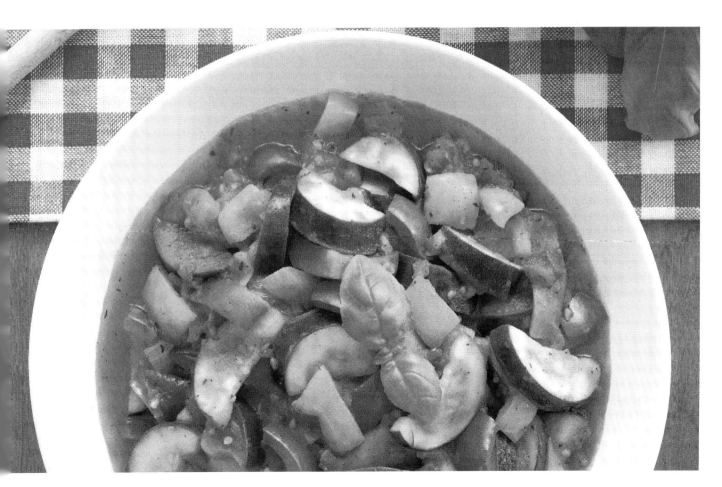

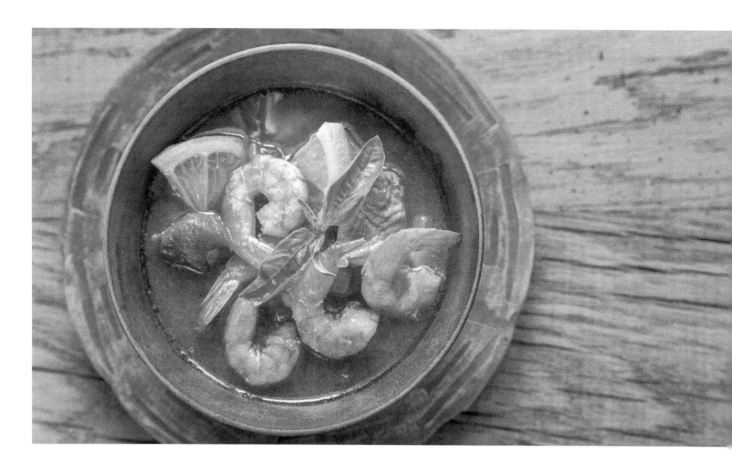

- **Variety at Hand**

From appetizers to main courses and desserts, a comprehensive Crock Pot Cookbook offers a multitude of options, ensuring you don't get stuck in a recipe rut.

- **Ingredient Guidance**

The cookbook can suggest which ingredients fare best in slow cooking, preventing potential culinary missteps.

- **Tailored Cooking Times**

Each recipe will have a specific cooking time, so you can plan when to start your Crock Pot to have a meal ready precisely when you want it.

- **Cost-Efficient Meals**

Many Crock Pot recipes can transform less expensive ingredients (like tougher cuts of meat) into gourmet dishes, and a good cookbook will provide plenty of these economical options.

- **Tips and Tricks**

Beyond just recipes, the cookbook can offer tips for getting the most out of your Crock Pot, from optimal layering of ingredients to maintenance and cleaning hacks.

- **Portion Guidance**

Whether you're cooking for a couple or a large family gathering, the cookbook can provide recipes suitable for different group sizes, reducing guesswork.

- **Nutritional Information**

For those mindful of their health, many cookbooks include nutritional info, helping users make informed dietary choices.

## Some tips for Crock Pot

**Layer wisely:** Heavier ingredients like root vegetables should go on the bottom because they take longer to cook. Meats are usually next, followed by softer vegetables and herbs.

**Avoid Overfilling:** A good rule of thumb is to fill the Crock Pot no more than two-thirds full to ensure even cooking and prevent spillage.

**Thaw before cooking:** Frozen ingredients will affect cooking times and may not reach safe temperatures quickly enough. It is best to thaw frozen meat and vegetables completely before adding them.

**Less flipping:** Every time the lid is lifted, heat and steam are released, which can significantly increase cooking time. Only turn on when necessary, such as stirring or checking doneness.

**Use the correct size:** If you're halving a recipe, use a smaller pan. If the pot is too large for the amount of food, it may cook faster and may burn.

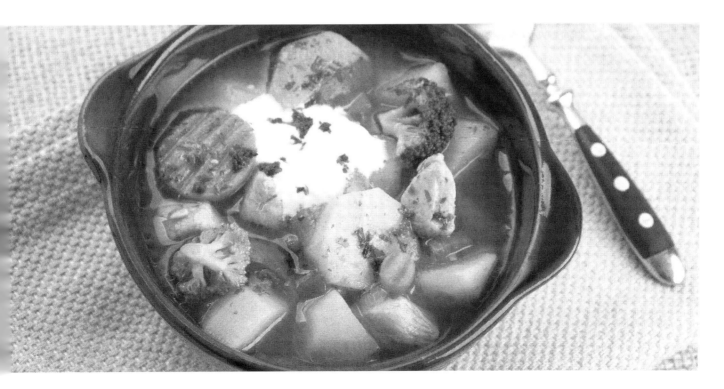

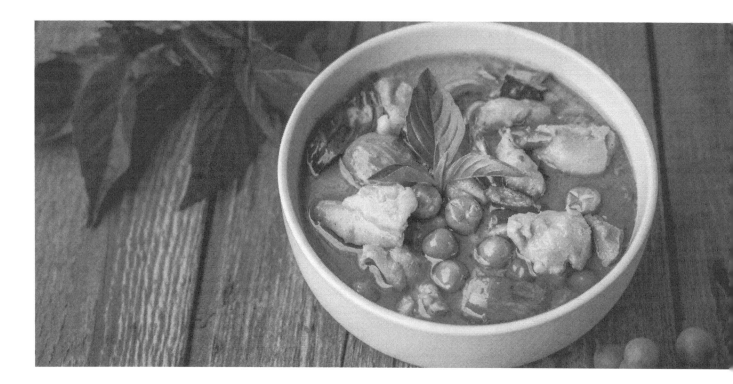

**Preheat your slow cooker:** Just like preheating your oven, turning your slow cooker on and letting it prehea while you're prepping can lead to more consistent cooking results.

**Choose Gradual Heat:** If a recipe calls for you to switch from a "low" setting to a "high" setting, let the cooke adjust gradually. Sudden changes may crack the ceramic insert.

**Be careful with dairy:** Dairy products such as milk, cream, and soft cheeses can curdle if added too early in the slow-cooking process. It is best to add them in the last hour of cooking.

**Reduce Fat:** Too much fat can lead to greasy results. Remove much of the fat from meat, and consider skim ming the fat from the top before serving.

**Spices and Herbs:** Dried herbs and spices become more potent in slow cooking, so adjust accordingly. Howev er, fresh herbs may lose their flavor during prolonged cooking, so it's best to add them near the end.

**Liquid Does Not Evaporate:** Unlike traditional stovetop cooking, liquid in a slow cooker does not decrease. I using a traditional recipe, reduce the amount of liquid. But always make sure there is enough liquid to cover th bottom to avoid burning.

**Even Heat:** For even heat and to avoid hot spots, rotate the insert half a turn every hour, especially with olde models that do not have consistent heating elements.

**Cleaning Tip:** To make cleaning easier, you can use a slow cooker liner or lightly grease the inside of the inse before adding ingredients.

With these tips, you can maximize your Crock Pot's efficiency, safety, and cooking potential. Happy slow cook ing!

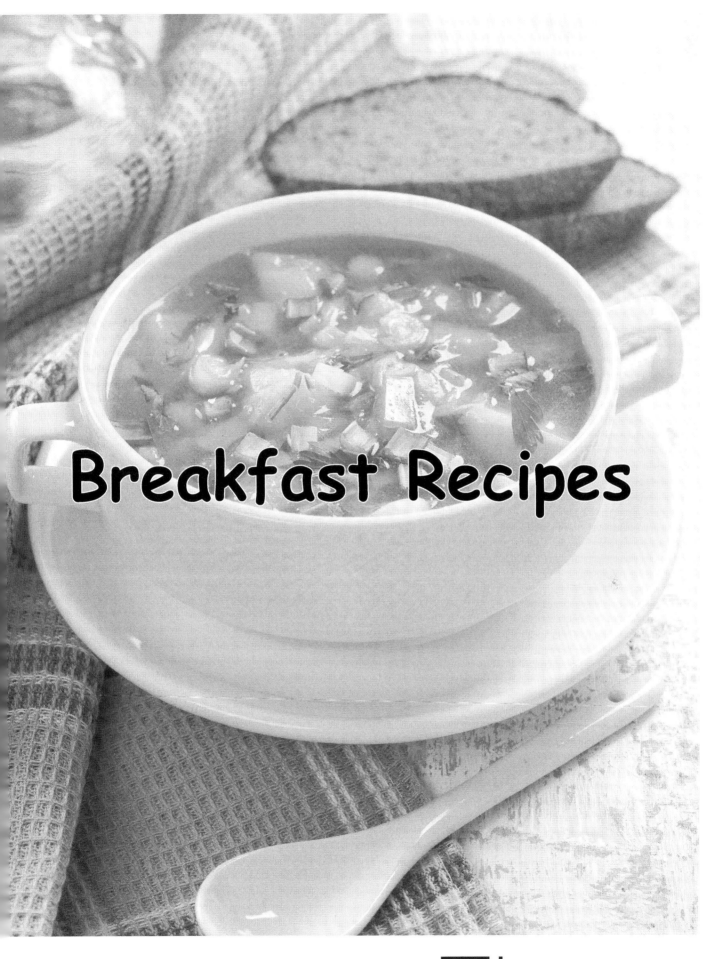

# Breakfast Recipes

# Breakfast Recipes

## Chicken Cabbage Medley

Servings: 5 | Cooking Time: 4.5 Hrs

**Ingredients:**
- 6 oz. ground chicken
- 10 oz. cabbage, chopped
- 1 white onion, sliced
- ½ cup tomato juice
- 1 tsp sugar
- ½ tsp salt
- 1 tsp ground black pepper
- 4 tbsp chicken stock
- 2 garlic cloves

**Directions:**
1. Whisk tomato juice with black pepper, salt, sugar, and chicken stock in a bowl.
2. Spread the onion slices, chicken, and cabbage in the Crock Pot.
3. Pour the tomato-stock mixture over the veggies and top with garlic cloves.
4. Put the cooker's lid on and set the cooking time to 4 hours 30 minutes on High settings.
5. Serve.

**Nutrition Info:**
- Info Per Serving: Calories 91, Total Fat 3.1g, Fiber 2g, Total Carbs 9.25g, Protein 8g

## Cranberry Oatmeal

Servings: 4 | Cooking Time: 8 Hours 15 Minutes

**Ingredients:**
- 1 cup dried cranberries
- 1 cup steel cut oats
- 1 cup dates, chopped
- 4 cups water
- 2 tablespoons honey
- ½ cup half and half

**Directions:**
1. Grease a crockpot and add all the ingredients except the half and half and honey.
2. Cover and cook on LOW for about 8 hours.
3. Stir in honey and half and half and dish out to serve.

**Nutrition Info:**
- Info Calories: 289 Fat: 5g Carbohydrates: 59.7g

## Quinoa Breakfast Bars

Servings: 8 | Cooking Time: 4 Hours

**Ingredients:**
- 2 tablespoons maple syrup
- 2 tablespoons almond butter, melted
- Cooking spray
- ½ teaspoon cinnamon powder
- 1 cup almond milk
- 2 eggs
- ½ cup raisins
- 1/3 cup quinoa
- 1/3 cup almonds, roasted and chopped
- 1/3 cup dried apples, chopped
- 2 tablespoons chia seeds

**Directions:**
1. In a bowl, mix almond butter with maple syrup, cinnamon, milk, eggs, quinoa, raisins, almonds, apples and chia seeds and stir really well.
2. Grease your Crock Pot with the spray, line it with parchment paper, spread quinoa mix, cover and cook on Low for 4 hours.
3. Leave mix aside to cool down, slice and serve for breakfast.

**Nutrition Info:**
- Info calories 300, fat 7, fiber 8, carbs 22, protein 5

# Raspberry Chia Porridge

Servings:4 | Cooking Time: 4 Hours

**Ingredients:**
- 1 cup raspberry
- 3 tablespoons maple syrup
- 1 cup chia seeds
- 4 cups of milk

**Directions:**
1. Put chia seeds and milk in the Crock Pot and cook the mixture on low for 4 hours.
2. Meanwhile, mix raspberries and maple syrup in the blender and blend the mixture until smooth.
3. When the chia porridge is cooked, transfer it in the serving bowls and top with blended raspberry mixture.

**Nutrition Info:**
InfoPer Serving: 315 calories, 13.1g protein, 37.7g carbohydrates, 13.9g fat, 11.7g fiber, 20mg cholesterol, 121mg sodium, 332mg potassium

# Berry-berry Jam

Servings: 6 | Cooking Time: 4 Hrs

**Ingredients:**
- 1 cup white sugar
- 1 cup strawberries
- 1 tbsp gelatin
- 3 tbsp water
- 1 tbsp lemon zest
- 1 tsp lemon juice
- ½ cup blueberries

**Directions:**
1. Take a blender jug and add berries, sugar, lemon juice, and lemon zest to puree.
2. Blend this blueberry-strawberry mixture for 3 minutes until smooth.
3. Pour this berry mixture into the base of your Crock Pot.
4. Put the cooker's lid on and set the cooking time to 1 hour on High settings.
5. Mix gelatin with 3 tbsp water in a bowl and pour it into the berry mixture.
6. Again, put the cooker's lid on and set the cooking time to 3 hours on High settings.
7. Allow the jam to cool down.
8. Serve.

**Nutrition Info:**
Info Per Serving: Calories 163, Total Fat 8.3g, Fiber 2g, Total Carbs 20.48g, Protein 3g

# Sweet Pepper Boats

Servings: 4 | Cooking Time: 3 Hrs

**Ingredients:**
- 2 red sweet pepper, cut in half
- 7 oz. ground chicken
- 5 oz. Parmesan, cubed
- 1 tbsp sour cream
- 1 tbsp flour
- 1 egg
- 2 tsp almond milk
- 1 tsp salt
- ½ tsp ground black pepper
- ¼ tsp butter

**Directions:**
1. Take the ground chicken in a large bowl.
2. Stir in sour cream, flour, almond milk, butter, whisked eggs, and black pepper.
3. Mix well and divide this chicken mixture in the sweet peppers.
4. Top each stuffed pepper with cheese cube.
5. Put the cooker's lid on and set the cooking time to 3 hours on High settings.
6. Serve warm.

**Nutrition Info:**
Info Per Serving: Calories 261, Total Fat 8.9g, Fiber 1g, Total Carbs 19.15g, Protein 26g

# Nutmeg Squash Oatmeal

Servings: 6 | Cooking Time: 8 Hrs

**Ingredients:**
- ½ cup almonds, soaked for 12 hours in water and drained
- ½ cup walnuts, chopped
- 2 apples, peeled, cored and cubed
- 1 butternut squash, peeled and cubed
- ½ tsp nutmeg, ground
- 1 tsp cinnamon powder
- 1 tbsp sugar
- 1 cup milk

**Directions:**
1. Toss almond with apples, walnuts, nutmeg, sugar, squash, and cinnamon in the base of your Crock Pot.
2. Pour in milk and give it a gentle stir.
3. Put the cooker's lid on and set the cooking time to 8 hours on Low settings.
4. Serve.

**Nutrition Info:**
- Info Per Serving: Calories 178, Total Fat 7g, Fiber 7g, Total Carbs 9g, Protein 4g

# Carrot Oatmeal

Servings:4 | Cooking Time: 6 Hours

**Ingredients:**
- 1 cup oatmeal
- 1 cup carrot, shredded
- 1 tablespoon raisins
- 1 tablespoon maple syrup
- 2 cups of water
- 1 teaspoon butter

**Directions:**
1. Put all ingredients in the Crock Pot.
2. Close the lid and cook the oatmeal on low for 6 hours.
3. Carefully mix the cooked meal.

**Nutrition Info:**
- InfoPer Serving: 117 calories, 3g protein, 21.7g carbohydrates, 2.g fat, 2.8g fiber, 3mg cholesterol, 31mg sodium, 191mg potassium

# Zucchini And Cauliflower Eggs Mix

Servings: 2 | Cooking Time: 6 Hours

**Ingredients:**
- 2 spring onions, chopped
- A pinch of salt and black pepper
- 4 eggs, whisked
- ½ cup cauliflower florets
- 1 zucchini, grated
- ¼ cup cheddar cheese, shredded
- ¼ cup whipping cream
- 1 tablespoon chives, chopped
- Cooking spray

**Directions:**
1. Grease the Crock Pot with the cooking spray and mix the eggs with the spring onions, cauliflower and the other ingredient inside.
2. Put the lid on and cook on Low for 6 hours.
3. Divide the mix between plates and serve for breakfast.

**Nutrition Info:**
- Info calories 211, fat 7, fiber 4, carbs 5, protein 5

# Creamy Breakfast

Servings: 1 | Cooking Time: 3 Hours

**Ingredients:**
- 1 teaspoon cinnamon powder
- ½ teaspoon nutmeg, ground
- ½ cup almonds, chopped
- 1 teaspoon sugar
- 1 and ½ cup heavy cream
- ¼ teaspoon cardamom, ground
- ¼ teaspoon cloves, ground

**Directions:**
1. In your Crock Pot, mix cream with cinnamon, nutmeg, almonds, sugar, cardamom and cloves, stir, cover, cook on Low for 3 hours, divide into bowls and serve for breakfast

**Nutrition Info:**
- Info calories 250, fat 12, fiber 4, carbs 8, protein 16

# Creamy Bacon Millet

Servings: 6 | Cooking Time: 4 Hrs 10 Minutes

**Ingredients:**
- 3 cup millet
- 6 cup chicken stock
- 1 tsp salt
- 4 tbsp heavy cream
- 5 oz. bacon, chopped

**Directions:**
1. Add millet and chicken stock to the Crock Pot.
2. Stir in chopped bacon and salt.
3. Put the cooker's lid on and set the cooking time to 4 hours on High settings.
4. Stir in cream and again cover the lid of the Crock Pot.
5. Cook for 10 minutes on High setting.
6. Serve.

**Nutrition Info:**
Info Per Serving: Calories 572, Total Fat 17.8g, Fiber 9g, Total Carbs 83.09g, Protein 20g

# Apricot Oatmeal

Servings:4 | Cooking Time: 4 Hours

**Ingredients:**
- 1 ½ cup oatmeal
- 1 cup of water
- 3 cups of milk
- 1 cup apricots, pitted, sliced
- 1 teaspoon butter

**Directions:**
1. Put oatmeal in the Crock Pot.
2. Add water, milk, and butter.
3. Close the lid and cook the mixture on high for 1 hour.
4. Then add apricots, carefully mix the oatmeal and close the lid.
5. Cook the meal on Low for 3 hours.

**Nutrition Info:**
InfoPer Serving: 235 calories, 10.5g protein, 34g carbohydrates, 7g fat, 3.9g fiber, 18mg cholesterol, 97mg sodium, 317mg po-assium

# Peach, Vanilla And Oats Mix

Servings: 2 | Cooking Time: 8 Hours

**Ingredients:**
- ½ cup steel cut oats
- 2 cups almond milk
- ½ cup peaches, pitted and roughly chopped
- ½ teaspoon vanilla extract
- 1 teaspoon cinnamon powder

**Directions:**
1. In your Crock Pot, mix the oats with the almond milk, peaches and the other ingredients, toss, put the lid on and cook on Low for 8 hours.
2. Divide into bowls and serve for breakfast right away.

**Nutrition Info:**
- Info calories 261, fat 5, fiber 8, carbs 18, protein 6

# Oats Granola

Servings: 8 | Cooking Time: 2 Hours

**Ingredients:**
- 5 cups old-fashioned rolled oats
- 1/3 cup coconut oil
- 2/3 cup honey
- ½ cup almonds, chopped
- ½ cup peanut butter
- 1 tablespoon vanilla
- 2 teaspoons cinnamon powder
- 1 cup craisins
- Cooking spray

**Directions:**
1. Grease your Crock Pot with cooking spray, add oats, oil, honey, almonds, peanut butter, vanilla, craisins and cinnamon, toss just a bit, cover and cook on High for 2 hours, stirring every 30 minutes.
2. Divide into bowls and serve for breakfast.

**Nutrition Info:**
- Info calories 200, fat 3, fiber 6, carbs 9, protein 4

# Huevos Rancheros

Servings: 2 | Cooking Time: 3 Hours 15 Minutes

**Ingredients:**
- 1 tablespoon butter
- ½ cup black beans
- 2 tablespoons guacamole
- ¼ teaspoon cumin powder
- ¼ cup light cream
- ½ red onion, thinly sliced
- 2 eggs
- ½ oz. Mexican blend cheese, shredded
- 2 tablespoons red enchilada sauce

**Directions:**
1. Put all the ingredients in a large bowl except guacamole and butter and mix thoroughly.
2. Put butter in the crockpot and stir in the mixed ingredients.
3. Cover and cook on LOW for about 3 hours.
4. Dish out and top with guacamole to serve.

**Nutrition Info:**
Info Calories: 264 Fat: 18g Carbohydrates: 15g

# Roasted Tomato Shakshuka

Servings:5 | Cooking Time: 4 Hours

**Ingredients:**
- 1 onion, chopped
- 1 bell pepper, seeded and chopped
- 1 ½ pounds cherry tomatoes
- ½ tablespoon cumin seeds
- 2 sprigs thyme leaves
- ¼ cup extra virgin olive oil
- 4 organic eggs
- Salt and pepper to taste
- 1 tablespoon parsley, chopped
- A pinch of cayenne pepper

**Directions:**
1. Place the onions, bell pepper, cherry tomatoes, cumin and thyme leaves in the food processor. Pulse until smooth.
2. Pour half of the olive oil in the CrockPot and pour the tomato mixture.
3. Break gently the eggs on top of the tomato mixture.
4. Season with salt and pepper to taste.
5. Close the lid and cook on high for 3 hours or on low for 4 hours.
6. An hour before the cooking time ends, pour in the remaining oil and sprinkle with parsley and cayenne pepper.
7. Close the lid and continue cooking for another hour or two.

**Nutrition Info:**
Info Calories per serving: 253; Carbohydrates: 9.5g; Protein: 27.5g; Fat: 12.8g; Sugar: 1.4g; Sodium: 371mg; Fiber: 4.7g

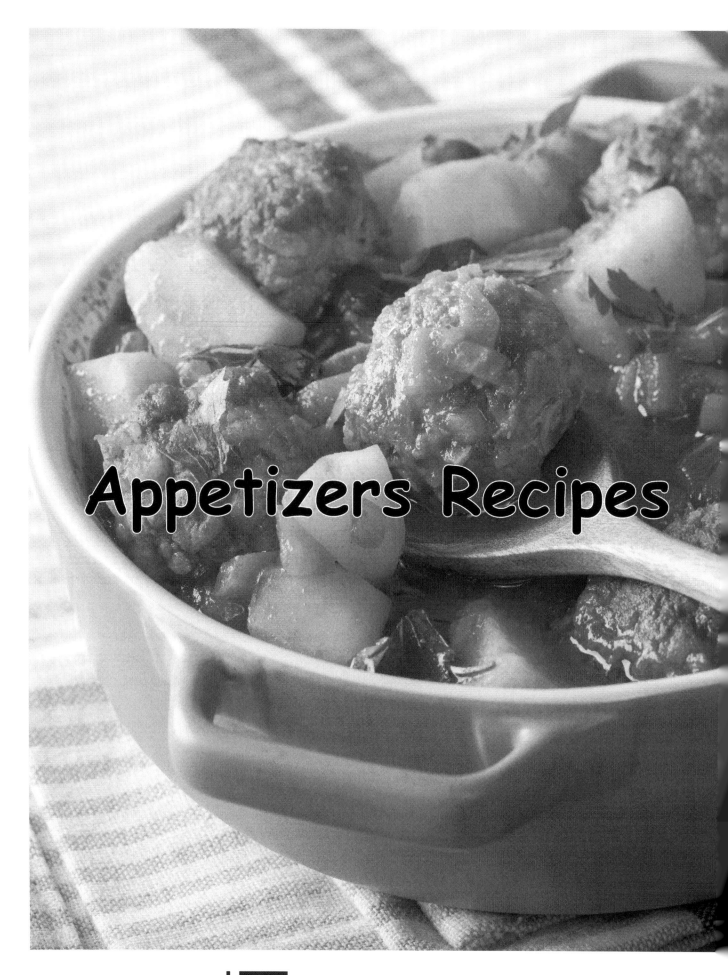

# Appetizers Recipes

# Appetizers Recipes

## Mozzarella Stuffed Meatballs

Servings: 8 | Cooking Time: 6 1/2 Hours

**Ingredients:**
- 2 pounds ground chicken
- 1 teaspoon dried basil
- 1/2 teaspoon dried oregano
- 1 egg
- 1/2 cup breadcrumbs
- Salt and pepper to taste
- Mini-mozzarella balls as needed
- 1/2 cup chicken stock

**Directions:**
1. Mix the ground chicken, basil, oregano, egg, breadcrumbs, salt and pepper in a bowl.
2. Take small pieces of the meat mixture and flatten it in your palm. Place a mozzarella ball in the center and gather the meat around the mozzarella.
3. Shape the meatballs, making sure they are well sealed and place them in a Crock Pot.
4. Add the chicken stock and cook on low settings for 6 hours.
5. Serve the meatballs warm or chilled.

## Spicy Glazed Pecans

Servings: 10 | Cooking Time: 3 1/4 Hours

**Ingredients:**
- 2 pounds pecans
- 1/2 cup butter, melted
- 1 teaspoon chili powder
- 1 teaspoon smoked paprika
- 1 teaspoon dried basil
- 1 teaspoon dried thyme
- 1/4 teaspoon cayenne pepper
- 1/2 teaspoon garlic powder
- 2 tablespoons honey

**Directions:**
1. Combine all the ingredients in your Crock Pot.
2. Mix well until all the ingredients are well distributed and the pecans are evenly glazed.
3. Cook on high settings for 3 hours.
4. Allow them to cool before serving.

## Stuffed Artichokes

Servings: 6 | Cooking Time: 6 1/2 Hours

**Ingredients:**
- 6 fresh artichokes
- 6 anchovy fillets, chopped
- 4 garlic cloves, minced
- 2 tablespoons olive oil
- 1 cup breadcrumbs
- 1 tablespoon chopped parsley
- Salt and pepper to taste
- 1/4 cup white wine

**Directions:**
1. Cut the stem of each artichoke so that it sits flat on your chopping board then cut the top off and trim the outer leaves, cleaning the center as well.
2. In a bowl, mix the anchovy fillets, garlic, olive oil, breadcrumbs and parsley. Add salt and pepper to taste.
3. Top each artichoke with breadcrumb mixture and rub it well into the leaves.
4. Place the artichokes in your Crock Pot and pour in the white wine.
5. Cook on low settings for 6 hours.
6. Serve the artichokes warm or chilled.

# Chili Corn Cheese Dip

Servings: 8 | Cooking Time: 2 1/4 Hours

**Ingredients:**
- 1 pound ground beef
- 2 tablespoons olive oil
- 1 shallot, chopped
- 1 can sweet corn, drained
- 1 can kidney beans, drained
- 1/2 cup beef stock
- 1 cup diced tomatoes
- 1/2 cup black olives, pitted and chopped
- 1 teaspoon dried oregano
- 1/2 teaspoon chili powder
- 1/2 teaspoon cumin powder
- 1/4 teaspoon garlic powder
- 2 cups grated Cheddar cheese
- Tortilla chips for serving

**Directions:**
1. Heat the oil in a skillet and stir in the ground beef. Cook for 5-7 minutes, stirring often.
2. Transfer the meat in a Crock Pot and add the remaining ingredients.
3. Add salt and pepper to taste and cover with its lid.
4. Cook on high settings for 2 hours.
5. Serve the dip warm with tortilla chips.

# Pork Ham Dip

Servings: 20 | Cooking Time: 6 1/4 Hours

**Ingredients:**
- 2 cups diced ham
- 1 pound ground pork
- 1 shallot, chopped
- 2 garlic cloves, chopped
- 1 teaspoon Dijon mustard
- 1 cup tomato sauce
- 1/2 cup chili sauce
- 1/2 cup cranberry sauce
- Salt and pepper to taste

**Directions:**
1. Heat a skillet over medium flame and add the ground pork. Cook for 5 minutes, stirring often.
2. Transfer the ground pork in a Crock Pot and add the remaining ingredients.
3. Adjust the taste with salt and pepper and cook on low settings for 6 hours.
4. Serve the dip warm or chilled.

# Nacho Sauce

Servings: 12 | Cooking Time: 6 1/4 Hours

**Ingredients:**
- 2 pounds ground beef
- 2 tablespoons Mexican seasoning
- 1 teaspoon chili powder
- 1 can diced tomatoes
- 2 shallots, chopped
- 4 garlic cloves, minced
- 1 can sweet corn, drained
- 2 cups grated Cheddar cheese

**Directions:**
1. Combine all the ingredients in your Crock Pot.
2. Cook on low settings for 6 hours.
3. This dip is best served warm.

# Goat Cheese Stuffed Mushrooms

Servings: 6 | Cooking Time: 4 1/4 Hours

**Ingredients:**
- 12 medium size mushrooms
- 6 oz. goat cheese
- 1 egg
- 1/2 cup breadcrumbs
- 1 poblano pepper, chopped
- 1 teaspoon dried oregano

**Directions:**
1. Mix the goat cheese, egg, breadcrumbs, pepper and oregano in a bowl.
2. Stuff each mushroom with the goat cheese mixture and place them all in a Crock Pot.
3. Cover the pot and cook on low settings for 4 hours.
4. Serve the mushrooms warm or chilled.

# Swiss Cheese Fondue

Servings: 10 | Cooking Time: 4 1/4 Hours

**Ingredients:**
- 1 garlic cloves
- 2 cups dry white wine
- 2 cups grated Swiss cheese
- 1 cup grated Cheddar
- 2 tablespoons cornstarch
- 1 pinch nutmeg

**Directions:**
1. Rub the inside of your Crock Pot with a garlic clove. Discard the clove once done.
2. Add the remaining ingredients and cook on low heat for 4 hours.
3. Serve the fondue warm with vegetable sticks, croutons or pretzels.

# Zesty Lamb Meatballs

Servings: 10 | Cooking Time: 7 1/4 Hours

**Ingredients:**
- 3 pounds ground lamb
- 1 shallot, chopped
- 2 garlic cloves, minced
- 1 tablespoon lemon zest
- 1/4 teaspoon five-spice powder
- 1/2 teaspoon cumin powder
- 1/4 teaspoon cumin powder
- 1/4 teaspoon chili powder
- 1/2 cup raisins, chopped
- 1 teaspoon dried mint
- Salt and pepper to taste
- 2 cups tomato sauce
- 1 lemon, juiced
- 1 bay leaf
- 1 thyme sprig
- 1 red chili, chopped

**Directions:**
1. Mix the tomato sauce, lemon juice, bay leaf, thyme sprig and red chili in your Crock Pot.
2. Combine the remaining ingredients in a bowl and mix well. Season with salt and pepper and give it a good mix.
3. Form small balls and place them in the sauce.
4. Cover with its lid and cook on low settings for 7 hours.
5. Serve the meatballs warm or chilled.

# Bacon Wrapped Dates

Servings: 8 | Cooking Time: 1 3/4 Hours

**Ingredients:**
- 16 dates, pitted
- 16 almonds
- 16 slices bacon

**Directions:**
1. Stuff each date with an almond.
2. Wrap each date in bacon and place the wrapped dates in your Crock Pot.
3. Cover with its lid and cook on high settings for 1 1/4 hours.
4. Serve warm or chilled.

# Chipotle Bbq Meatballs

Servings: 10 | Cooking Time: 7 1/2 Hours

**Ingredients:**
- 3 pounds ground pork
- 2 garlic cloves, minced
- 2 shallots, chopped
- 2 chipotle peppers, chopped
- Salt and pepper to taste
- 2 cups BBQ sauce
- 1/4 cup cranberry sauce
- 1 bay leaf

**Directions:**
1. Mix the ground pork, garlic, shallots, chipotle peppers, salt and pepper in a bowl.
2. Combine the BBQ sauce, cranberry sauce, bay leaf, salt and pepper in your Crock Pot.
3. Form small meatballs and drop them in the sauce.
4. Cover the pot with its lid and cook on low settings for 7 hours.
5. Serve the meatballs warm or chilled with cocktail skewers or toothpicks.

# Cheesy Chicken Bites

Servings: 10 | Cooking Time: 6 1/4 Hours

**Ingredients:**
- 4 chicken breasts, cut into bite-size cubes
- 1/4 cup all-purpose flour
- Salt and pepper to taste
- 1 cup cream cheese
- 2 roasted red bell peppers
- 1 cup shredded mozzarella
- 1/4 teaspoon chili powder

**Directions:**
1. Mix the cream cheese, bell peppers, chili powder, salt and pepper in a blender and pulse until smooth.
2. Pour the mixture in your Crock Pot and add the remaining ingredients.
3. Cook on low settings for 6 hours.
4. Serve the chicken bites warm or chilled.

# Artichoke Dip

Servings: 20 | Cooking Time: 6 1/4 Hours

**Ingredients:**
- 2 sweet onions, chopped
- 1 red chili, chopped
- 2 garlic cloves, chopped
- 1 jar artichoke hearts, drained and chopped
- 1 cup cream cheese
- 1 cup heavy cream
- 2 oz. blue cheese, crumbled
- 2 tablespoons chopped cilantro

**Directions:**
1. Mix the onions, chili, garlic, artichoke hearts, cream cheese, heavy cream and blue cheese in a Crock Pot.
2. Cook on low settings for 6 hours.
3. When done, stir in the cilantro and serve the dip warm or chilled.

# Cheeseburger Dip

Servings: 20 | Cooking Time: 6 1/4 Hours

**Ingredients:**
- 2 pounds ground beef
- 1 tablespoon canola oil
- 2 sweet onions, chopped
- 4 garlic cloves, chopped
- 1/2 cup tomato sauce
- 1 tablespoon Dijon mustard
- 2 tablespoons pickle relish
- 1 cup shredded processed cheese
- 1 cup grated Cheddar

**Directions:**
1. Heat the canola oil in a skillet and stir in the ground beef. Sauté for 5 minutes then add the meat in your Crock Pot.
2. Stir in the remaining ingredients and cover with the pot's lid.
3. Cook on low settings for 6 hours.
4. The dip is best served warm.

# Molasses Lime Meatballs

Servings: 10 | Cooking Time: 8 1/4 Hours

**Ingredients:**
- 3 pounds ground beef
- 2 garlic cloves, minced
- 1 shallot, chopped
- 1/2 cup oat flour
- 1/2 teaspoon cumin powder
- 1/2 teaspoon chili powder
- 1 egg
- Salt and pepper to taste
- 1/2 cup molasses
- 1/4 cup soy sauce
- 2 tablespoons lime juice
- 1/2 cup beef stock
- 1 tablespoon Worcestershire sauce

**Directions:**
1. Combine the molasses, soy sauce, lime juice, stock and Worcestershire sauce in your Crock Pot.
2. In a bowl, mix the ground beef, garlic, shallot, oat flour, cumin powder, chili powder, egg, salt and pepper and mix well.
3. Form small balls and place them in the sauce.
4. Cover the pot and cook on low settings for 8 hours.
5. Serve the meatballs warm or chilled.

# Asian Marinated Mushrooms

Servings: 8 | Cooking Time: 8 1/4 Hours

**Ingredients:**
- 2 pounds mushrooms
- 1 cup soy sauce
- 1 cup water
- 1/2 cup brown sugar
- 1/4 cup rice vinegar
- 1/2 teaspoon chili powder

**Directions:**
1. Combine all the ingredients in your Crock Pot.
2. Cover the crock pot and cook on low settings for 8 hours.
3. Allow to cool in the pot before serving.

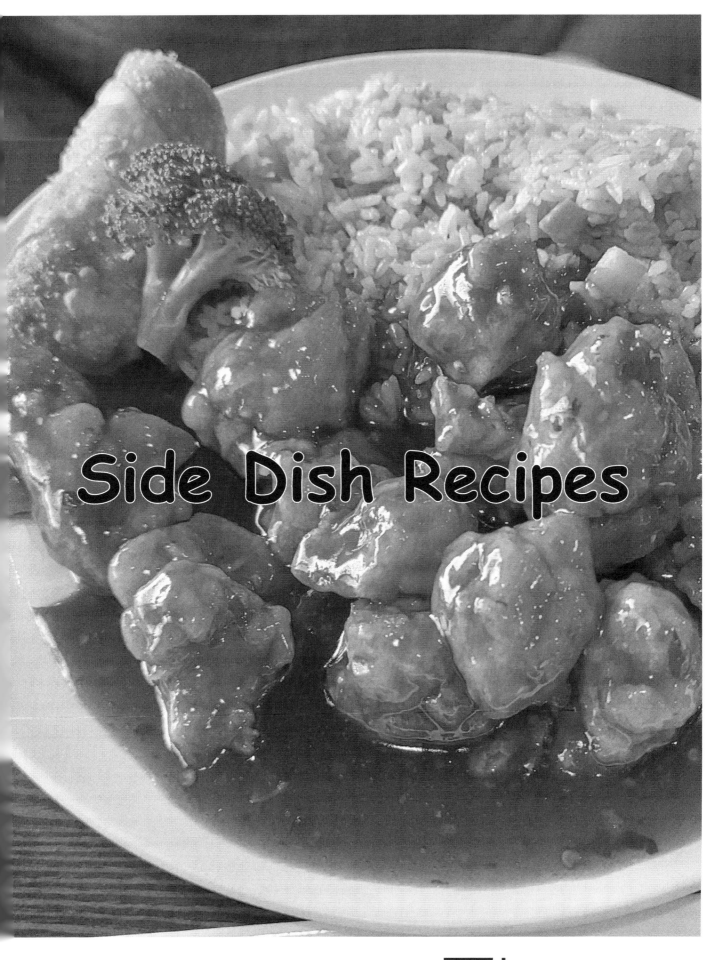

# Side Dish Recipes

# Side Dish Recipes

## Cauliflower And Carrot Gratin

Servings: 12 | Cooking Time: 7 Hours

**Ingredients:**
- 16 ounces baby carrots
- 6 tablespoons butter, soft
- 1 cauliflower head, florets separated
- Salt and black pepper to the taste
- 1 yellow onion, chopped
- 1 teaspoon mustard powder
- 1 and ½ cups milk
- 6 ounces cheddar cheese, grated
- ½ cup breadcrumbs

**Directions:**
1. Put the butter in your Crock Pot, add carrots, cauliflower, onion, salt, pepper, mustard powder and milk and toss.
2. Sprinkle cheese and breadcrumbs all over, cover and cook on Low for 7 hours.
3. Divide between plates and serve as a side dish.

**Nutrition Info:**
- Info calories 182, fat 4, fiber 7, carbs 9, protein 4

## Veggie And Garbanzo Mix

Servings: 4 | Cooking Time: 6 Hours

**Ingredients:**
- 15 ounces canned garbanzo beans, drained
- 3 cups cauliflower florets
- 1 cup green beans
- 1 cup carrot, sliced
- 14 ounces veggie stock
- ½ cup onion, chopped
- 2 teaspoons curry powder
- ¼ cup basil, chopped
- 14 ounces coconut milk

**Directions:**
1. In your Crock Pot, mix beans with cauliflower, green beans, carrot, onion, stock, curry powder, basil and milk, stir, cover and cook on Low for 6 hours.
2. Stir veggie mix again, divide between plates and serve as a side dish.

**Nutrition Info:**
- Info calories 219, fat 5, fiber 8, carbs 32, protein 7

## Coconut Bok Choy

Servings: 2 | Cooking Time: 1 Hour

**Ingredients:**
- 1 pound bok choy, torn
- ½ cup chicken stock
- ½ teaspoon chili powder
- 1 garlic clove, minced
- 1 teaspoon ginger, grated
- 1 tablespoon coconut oil
- Salt to the taste

**Directions:**
1. In your Crock Pot, mix the bok choy with the stock and the other ingredients, toss, put the lid on and cook on High for 1 hour.
2. Divide between plates and serve as a side dish.

**Nutrition Info:**
- Info calories 100, fat 1, fiber 2, carbs 7, protein 4

# Farro Rice Pilaf

Servings: 12 | Cooking Time: 5 Hours

**Ingredients:**
- 1 shallot, chopped
- 1 tsp garlic, minced
- A drizzle of olive oil
- 1 and ½ cups whole grain farro
- ¾ cup wild rice
- 6 cups chicken stock
- Salt and black pepper to the taste
- 1 tbsp parsley and sage, chopped
- ½ cup hazelnuts, toasted and chopped
- ¾ cup cherries, dried

**Directions:**
1. Add farro, rice, stock, and rest of the ingredients to the Crock Pot.
2. Put the cooker's lid on and set the cooking time to 5 hours on Low settings.
3. Serve warm.

**Nutrition Info:**
Info Per Serving: Calories: 120, Total Fat: 2g, Fiber: 7g, Total Carbs: 20g, Protein: 3g

# Cider Dipped Farro

Servings: 6 | Cooking Time: 5 Hours

**Ingredients:**
- 1 tbsp apple cider vinegar
- 1 cup whole-grain farro
- 1 tsp lemon juice
- Salt to the taste
- 3 cups of water
- 1 tbsp olive oil
- ½ cup cherries, dried and chopped
- ¼ cup green onions, chopped
- 10 mint leaves, chopped
- 2 cups cherries, pitted and halved

**Directions:**
1. Add water and farro to the Crock Pot.
2. Put the cooker's lid on and set the cooking time to 5 hours on Low settings.
3. Toss the cooker farro with salt, cherries, mint, green onion, lemon juice, and oil in a bowl.
4. Serve fresh.

**Nutrition Info:**
Info Per Serving: Calories: 162, Total Fat: 3g, Fiber: 6g, Total Carbs: 12g, Protein: 4g

# Spinach And Squash Side Salad

Servings: 12 | Cooking Time: 4 Hours

**Ingredients:**
- 3 pounds butternut squash, peeled and cubed
- 1 yellow onion, chopped
- 2 teaspoons thyme, chopped
- 3 garlic cloves, minced
- A pinch of salt and black pepper
- 10 ounces veggie stock
- 6 ounces baby spinach

**Directions:**
1. In your Crock Pot, mix squash cubes with onion, thyme, salt, pepper and stock, stir, cover and cook on Low for 4 hours.
2. Transfer squash mix to a bowl, add spinach, toss, divide between plates and serve as a side dish.

**Nutrition Info:**
Info calories 100, fat 1, fiber 4, carbs 18, protein 4

# Beans, Carrots And Spinach Salad

Servings: 6 | Cooking Time: 7 Hours

**Ingredients:**
- 1 and ½ cups northern beans
- 1 yellow onion, chopped
- 5 carrots, chopped
- 2 garlic cloves, minced
- ½ teaspoon oregano, dried
- Salt and black pepper to the taste
- 4 and ½ cups chicken stock
- 5 ounces baby spinach
- 2 teaspoons lemon peel, grated
- 1 avocado, peeled, pitted and chopped
- 3 tablespoons lemon juice
- ¾ cup feta cheese, crumbled
- 1/3 cup pistachios, chopped

**Directions:**
1. In your Crock Pot, mix beans with onion, carrots, garlic, oregano, salt, pepper and stock, stir, cover and cook on Low for ⁷ hours.
2. Drain beans and veggies, transfer them to a salad bowl, add baby spinach, lemon peel, avocado, lemon juice, pistachios and cheese, toss, divide between plates and serve as a side dish.

**Nutrition Info:**
- Info calories 300, fat 8, fiber 14, carbs 43, protein 16

# Mashed Potatoes

Servings: 2 | Cooking Time: 6 Hours

**Ingredients:**
- 1 pound gold potatoes, peeled and cubed
- 2 garlic cloves, chopped
- 1 cup milk
- 1 cup water
- 2 tablespoons butter
- A pinch of salt and white pepper

**Directions:**
1. In your Crock Pot, mix the potatoes with the water, salt and pepper, put the lid on and cook on Low for 6 hours.
2. Mash the potatoes, add the rest of the ingredients, whisk and serve.

**Nutrition Info:**
- Info calories 135, fat 4, fiber 2, carbs 10, protein 4

# Cauliflower And Potatoes Mix

Servings: 2 | Cooking Time: 4 Hours

**Ingredients:**
- 1 cup cauliflower florets
- ½ pound sweet potatoes, peeled and cubed
- 1 cup veggie stock
- ½ cup tomato sauce
- 1 tablespoon chives, chopped
- Salt and black pepper to the taste
- 1 teaspoon sweet paprika

**Directions:**
1. In your Crock Pot, mix the cauliflower with the potatoes, stock and the other ingredients, toss, put the lid on and cook on High for 4 hours.
2. Divide between plates and serve as a side dish.

**Nutrition Info:**
- Info calories 135, fat 5, fiber 1, carbs 7, protein 3

# Tamale Side Dish

Servings: 5 | Cooking Time: 7 Hours

**Ingredients:**
- 12 oz. masa harina
- 1 cup chicken stock
- ½ tsp salt
- 1 tsp onion powder
- 1 onion, chopped
- 5 tbsp olive oil
- 5 corn husks
- 5 cups of water

**Directions:**
1. Chicken Mix masa harina with chicken salt, salt, onion powder.
2. Stir in the chopped onion, and olive oil, then knead this dough.
3. Soak corn husks for 15 minutes in water then drain.
4. Spread the corn husks on the working surface.
5. Divide the masa harina mixture over the corn husks.
6. Roll the corn husk around the filling, then place these rolls in the Crock Pot.
7. Put the cooker's lid on and set the cooking time to 7 hours on Low settings.
8. Serve fresh.

**Nutrition Info:**
Info Per Serving: Calories: 214, Total Fat: 14.8g, Fiber: 2g, Total Carbs: 18g, Protein: 3g

# Berry Wild Rice

Servings: 4 | Cooking Time: 5 Hours 30 Minutes

**Ingredients:**
- 2 cups wild rice
- 4 cups of water
- 1 tsp salt
- 6 oz. cherries, dried
- 1 tbsp chives
- 1 tbsp butter
- 2 tbsp heavy cream

**Directions:**
1. Add wild rice, salt, water, and dried cherries to the Crock Pot.
2. Put the cooker's lid on and set the cooking time to 5 hours on High settings.
3. Stir in cream and butter, then cover again to cook for 30 minutes on the low setting.
4. Serve.

**Nutrition Info:**
Info Per Serving: Calories: 364, Total Fat: 6.6g, Fiber: 6g, Total Carbs: 66.97g, Protein: 12g

# Okra Side Dish(1)

Servings: 4 | Cooking Time: 3 Hours

**Ingredients:**
- 2 cups okra, sliced
- 1 and ½ cups red onion, roughly chopped
- 1 cup cherry tomatoes, halved
- 2 and ½ cups zucchini, sliced
- 2 cups red and yellow bell peppers, sliced
- 1 cup white mushrooms, sliced
- ½ cup olive oil
- ½ cup balsamic vinegar
- 2 tablespoons basil, chopped
- 1 tablespoon thyme, chopped

**Directions:**
1. In your Crock Pot, mix okra with onion, tomatoes, zucchini, bell peppers, mushrooms, basil and thyme.
2. In a bowl mix oil with vinegar, whisk well, add to the Crock Pot, cover and cook on High for 3 hours.
3. Divide between plates and serve as a side dish.

**Nutrition Info:**
- Info calories 233, fat 12, fiber 4, carbs 8, protein 4

# Mustard Brussels Sprouts

Servings: 2 | Cooking Time: 3 Hours

**Ingredients:**
- ½ pounds Brussels sprouts, trimmed and halved
- A pinch of salt and black pepper
- 2 tablespoons mustard
- ½ cup veggie stock
- 1 tablespoons olive oil
- 2 tablespoons maple syrup
- 1 tablespoon thyme, chopped

**Directions:**
1. In your Crock Pot, mix the sprouts with the mustard and the other ingredients, toss, put the lid on and cook on Low for hours.
2. Divide between plates and serve as a side dish.

**Nutrition Info:**
- Info calories 170, fat 4, fiber 4, carbs 14, protein 6

# Kale Mix

Servings: 2 | Cooking Time: 2 Hours

**Ingredients:**
- 1 pound baby kale
- ½ tablespoon tomato paste
- ½ cup chicken stock
- ½ teaspoon chili powder
- A pinch of salt and black pepper
- 1 tablespoon olive oil
- 1 small yellow onion, chopped
- 1 tablespoon apple cider vinegar

**Directions:**
1. In your Crock Pot, mix the kale with the tomato paste, stock and the other ingredients, toss, put the lid on and cook on Low for 2 hours.
2. Divide between plates and serve as a side dish.

**Nutrition Info:**
- Info calories 200, fat 4, fiber 7, carbs 10, protein 3

# Garlicky Black Beans

Servings: 8 | Cooking Time: 7 Hours

**gredients:**
1 cup black beans, soaked overnight, drained and rinsed
1 cup of water
Salt and black pepper to the taste
1 spring onion, chopped
2 garlic cloves, minced
½ tsp cumin seeds

**rections:**
Add beans, salt, black pepper, cumin seeds, garlic, and onion to the Crock Pot.
Put the cooker's lid on and set the cooking time to 7 hours on Low settings.
Serve warm.

**utrition Info:**
Info Per Serving: Calories: 300, Total Fat: 4g, Fiber: 6g, Total Carbs: 20g, Protein: 15g

# Tarragon Sweet Potatoes

Servings: 4 | Cooking Time: 3 Hours

**gredients:**
1 pound sweet potatoes, peeled and cut into wedges
1 cup veggie stock
½ teaspoon chili powder
½ teaspoon cumin, ground
Salt and black pepper to the taste
1 tablespoon olive oil
1 tablespoon tarragon, dried
2 tablespoons balsamic vinegar

**irections:**
In your Crock Pot, mix the sweet potatoes with the stock, chili powder and the other ingredients, toss, put the lid on and cook
High for 3 hours.
Divide the mix between plates and serve as a side dish.

**utrition Info:**
Info calories 80, fat 4, fiber 4, carbs 8, protein 4

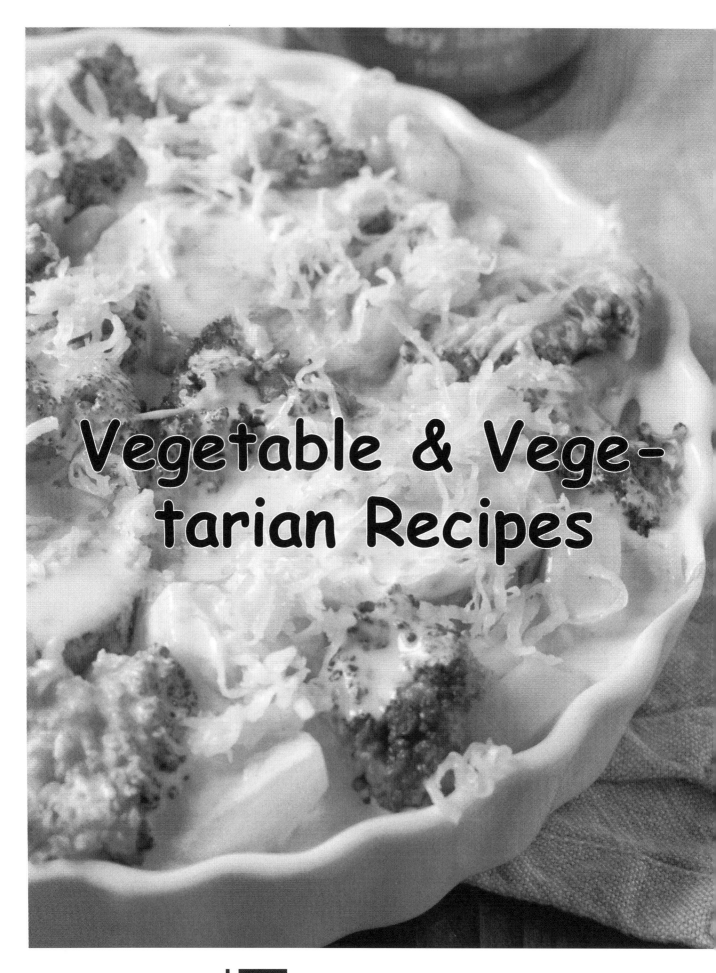

# Vegetable & Vegetarian Recipes

# Vegetable & Vegetarian Recipes

## Tofu Tikka Masala

Servings:4 | Cooking Time: 2 Hours

**Ingredients:**

- 1-pound tofu, cubed
- 1 teaspoon ground cumin
- 1 teaspoon garam masala
- ½ cup coconut cream
- 1 teaspoon minced garlic
- 1 teaspoon minced ginger
- 1 tablespoon lemon juice
- 1 tablespoon avocado oil

**Directions:**

1. In the mixing bowl mix avocado oil, lemon juice, minced ginger, garlic, coconut cream, garam masala, and ground cumin.
2. Then add tofu and carefully mix the mixture.
3. Leave it for 10 minutes and then transfer in the Crock Pot.
4. Close the lid and cook the meal on Low for 2 hours.

**Nutrition Info:**

InfoPer Serving: 159 calories, 10.2g protein, 4.6g carbohydrates, 12.5g fat, 2g fiber, 0mg cholesterol, 21mg sodium, 281mg potassium.

## Beet Salad

Servings:4 | Cooking Time: 5 Hours

**Ingredients:**

- 2 cups beet, peeled, chopped
- 3 oz goat cheese, crumbled
- 4 cups of water
- 1 tablespoon olive oil
- 1 teaspoon liquid honey
- 3 pecans, chopped

**Directions:**

1. Put beets in the Crock Pot.
2. Add water and cook them on high for 5 hours.
3. The drain water and transfer the cooked beets in the bowl.
4. Add olive oil, honey, and pecans. Shake the vegetables well and transfer them to the serving plates.
5. Top every serving with crumbled goat cheese.

**Nutrition Info:**

InfoPer Serving: 242 calories, 9.1g protein, 11.9g carbohydrates, 18.7g fat, 2.8g fiber, 22mg cholesterol, 146mg sodium, 16mg potassium.

## Mushroom Steaks

Servings:4 | Cooking Time: 2 Hours

**Ingredients:**

- 4 Portobello mushrooms
- 1 tablespoon avocado oil
- 1 tablespoon lemon juice
- 2 tablespoons coconut cream
- ½ teaspoon ground black pepper

**Directions:**

1. Slice Portobello mushrooms into steaks and sprinkle with avocado oil, lemon juice, coconut cream, and ground black pepper.
2. Then arrange the mushroom steaks in the Crock Pot in one layer (you will need to cook all mushroom steaks by 2 times).
3. Cook the meal on High for 1 hour.

**Nutrition Info:**

InfoPer Serving: 43 calories, 3.3g protein, 3.9g carbohydrates, 2.3g fat, 1.4g fiber, 0mg cholesterol, 2mg sodium, 339mg potassium.

# French Vegetable Stew

Servings: 6 | Cooking Time: 9 Hrs

**Ingredients:**
- 2 yellow onions, chopped
- 1 eggplant, sliced
- 4 zucchinis, sliced
- 2 garlic cloves, minced
- 2 green bell peppers, cut into medium strips
- 6 oz. canned tomato paste
- 2 tomatoes, cut into medium wedges
- 1 tsp oregano, dried
- 1 tsp sugar
- 1 tsp basil, dried
- Salt and black pepper to the taste
- 2 tbsp parsley, chopped
- ¼ cup olive oil
- A pinch of red pepper flakes, crushed

**Directions:**
1. Add onions, zucchinis, eggplant, garlic, tomato paste, bell peppers, sugar, basil, salt, black pepper, and oregano to the Crock Pot.
2. Put the cooker's lid on and set the cooking time to 9 hours on Low settings.
3. Stir in parsley and pepper flakes.
4. Serve warm.

**Nutrition Info:**
- Info Per Serving: Calories 269, Total Fat 7g, Fiber 6g, Total Carbs 17g, Protein 4g

# Eggplant Salad

Servings:5 | Cooking Time: 3 Hours

**Ingredients:**
- 4 eggplants, cubed
- 1 teaspoon salt
- 1 teaspoon ground black pepper
- 1 cup of water
- 1 tablespoon sesame oil
- 1 tablespoon apple cider vinegar
- 1 teaspoon sesame seeds
- 2 cups tomatoes, chopped

**Directions:**
1. Mix eggplants with salt and ground black pepper and leave for 10 minutes.
2. Then transfer the eggplants in the Crock Pot. Add water and cook them for 3 hours on High.
3. Drain water and cool the eggplants to the room temperature.
4. Add sesame oil, apple cider vinegar, sesame seeds, and tomatoes.
5. Gently shake the salad.

**Nutrition Info:**
- InfoPer Serving: 152 calories, 5.1g protein, 29g carbohydrates, 4g fat, 16.5g fiber, 0mg cholesterol, 479mg sodium, 1185m potassium.

# Beans Bake

Servings:4 | Cooking Time: 5 Hours

**Ingredients:**
1-pound green beans
1 tablespoon olive oil
1 teaspoon salt
½ teaspoon ground black pepper
2 tablespoons breadcrumbs
4 eggs, beaten

**Directions:**
1. Chop the green beans roughly and sprinkle them with salt and ground black pepper.
2. Then put them in the Crock Pot.
3. Sprinkle the vegetables with breadcrumbs and eggs.
4. Close the lid and cook the beans bake on Low for 5 hours.

**Nutrition Info:**
InfoPer Serving: 142 calories, 8.1g protein, 11g carbohydrates, 8.2g fat, 4.1g fiber, 164mg cholesterol, 675mg sodium, 306mg potassium.

# Stuffed Okra

Servings:4 | Cooking Time: 5 Hours

**Ingredients:**
1-pound okra
1 cup cauliflower, shredded
1 teaspoon curry powder
1 teaspoon tomato paste
- 1 teaspoon dried dill
- 1/3 cup coconut milk
- 1 tablespoon coconut oil

**Directions:**
1. Make the cuts in the okra and remove seeds.
2. Then mix shredded cauliflower with curry powder, tomato paste, and dried dill.
3. Fill every okra with cauliflower mixture and put in the Crock Pot.
4. Add coconut oil and coconut milk in the Crock Pot and close the lid.
5. Cook the okra on Low for 5 hours.

**Nutrition Info:**
InfoPer Serving: 130 calories, 3.3g protein, 11.6g carbohydrates, 8.5g fat, 5g fiber, 0mg cholesterol, 21mg sodium, 497mg potassium.

# Fragrant Appetizer Peppers

Servings:2 | Cooking Time: 1.5 Hours

**Ingredients:**
4 sweet peppers, seeded
¼ cup apple cider vinegar
1 red onion, sliced
1 teaspoon peppercorns
½ teaspoon sugar
¼ cup of water
1 tablespoon olive oil

**Directions:**
1. Slice the sweet peppers roughly and put in the Crock Pot.
2. Add all remaining ingredients and close the lid.
3. Cook the peppers on high for 1.5 hours.
4. Then cool the peppers well and store them in the fridge for up to 6 days.

**Nutrition Info:**
InfoPer Serving: 171 calories, 3.1g protein, 25.1g carbohydrates, 7.7g fat, 4.7g fiber, 0mg cholesterol, 11mg sodium, 564mg potassium.

# Vegetarian Red Coconut Curry

Servings:4 | Cooking Time: 3 Hours

**Ingredients:**
- 1 cup broccoli florets
- 1 large handful spinach, rinsed
- 1 tablespoon red curry paste
- 1 cup coconut cream
- 1 teaspoon garlic, minced

**Directions:**
1. Combine all ingredients in the crockpot.
2. Close the lid and cook on low for 3 hours or on high for 1 hour.

**Nutrition Info:**
- Info Calories per serving: 226; Carbohydrates: 8g; Protein: 5.2g; Fat:21.4 g; Sugar: 0.4g; Sodium: 341mg; Fiber:4.3 g

# Sautéed Greens

Servings:4 | Cooking Time: 1 Hour

**Ingredients:**
- 1 cup spinach, chopped
- 2 cups collard greens, chopped
- 1 cup Swiss chard, chopped
- 2 cups of water
- ½ cup half and half

**Directions:**
1. Put spinach, collard greens, and Swiss chard in the Crock Pot.
2. Add water and close the lid.
3. Cook the greens on High for 1 hour.
4. Then drain water and transfer the greens in the bowl.
5. Bring the half and half to boil and pour over greens.
6. Carefully mix the greens.

**Nutrition Info:**
- InfoPer Serving: 49 calories, 1.8g protein, 3.2g carbohydrates, 3.7g fat, 1.1g fiber, 11mg cholesterol, 45mg sodium, 117mg potassium.

# Sweet Potato And Lentils Pate

Servings:4 | Cooking Time: 6 Hours

**Ingredients:**
- 1 cup sweet potato, chopped
- ½ cup red lentils
- 2.5 cups water
- 1 tablespoon soy milk
- 1 teaspoon cayenne pepper
- ½ teaspoon salt

**Directions:**
1. Put all ingredients in the Crock Pot.
2. Close the lid and cook the mixture on low for 6 hours.
3. When the ingredients are cooked, transfer them in the blender and blend until smooth.
4. Put the cooked pate in the bowl and store it in the fridge for up to 4 days.

**Nutrition Info:**
- InfoPer Serving: 140 calories, 7.4g protein, 25.1g carbohydrates, 1.3g fat, 9.1g fiber, 3mg cholesterol, 322mg sodium, 488mg potassium.

# Sweet Potato Curry

Servings:4 | Cooking Time: 3.5 Hours

**Ingredients:**
- 2 cups sweet potatoes, chopped
- 1 cup spinach, chopped
- ½ onion, diced
- 1 teaspoon garlic, minced
- 1 teaspoon curry powder
- ½ teaspoon ground turmeric
- 1 tablespoon coconut oil
- 1 cup of coconut milk

**Directions:**
1. In the mixing bowl mix coconut milk, ground turmeric, curry powder, garlic, and pour it in the Crock Pot.
2. Add sweet potatoes, onion, and coconut oil.
3. Close the lid and cook the ingredients on High for 3 hours.
4. Then add spinach, carefully mix the mixture and cook it for 30 minutes on High.

**Nutrition Info:**
InfoPer Serving: 267 calories, 3g protein, 26.5g carbohydrates, 18g fat, 5.1g fiber, 0mg cholesterol, 23mg sodium, 849mg potassium.

# Miso Asparagus

Servings:2 | Cooking Time: 2.5 Hours

**Ingredients:**
- 1 teaspoon miso paste
- 1 cup of water
- 1 tablespoon fish sauce
- 10 oz asparagus, chopped
- 1 teaspoon avocado oil

**Directions:**
1. Mix miso paste with water and pour in the Crock Pot.
2. Add fish sauce, asparagus, and avocado oil.
3. Close the lid and cook the meal on High for 2.5 hours.

**Nutrition Info:**
InfoPer Serving: 40 calories, 3.9g protein, 6.7g carbohydrates, 0.6g fat, 3.2g fiber, 0mg cholesterol, 808mg sodium, 327mg potassium.

# Squash Noodles

Servings:4 | Cooking Time: 4 Hours

**Ingredients:**
- 1-pound butternut squash, seeded, halved
- 1 tablespoon vegan butter
- 1 teaspoon salt
- ½ teaspoon garlic powder
- 3 cups of water

**Directions:**
1. Pour water in the Crock Pot.
2. Add butternut squash and close the lid.
3. Cook the vegetable on high for 4 hours.
4. Then drain water and shred the squash flesh with the help of the fork and transfer in the bowl.
5. Add garlic powder, salt, and butter. Mix the squash noodles.

**Nutrition Info:**
InfoPer Serving: 78 calories, 1.2g protein, 13.5g carbohydrates, 3g fat, 2.3g fiber, 8mg cholesterol, 612mg sodium, 406mg potassium

Servings: 8 | Cooking Time: 6 Hrs

**Ingredients:**
- 2 sweet potatoes, peeled and sliced
- 2 red potatoes, peeled and sliced
- 6 oz. Parmesan, shredded
- 1 cup sweet corn
- 1 tsp salt
- 1 tsp paprika
- 1 tsp curry powder
- 2 red onions, sliced
- 1 cup flour
- 1 tsp baking soda
- ½ tsp apple cider vinegar
- 1 cup Greek Yogurt
- 3 tomatoes, sliced
- ¼ tsp butter

**Directions:**
1. Toss the vegetables with curry, salt, paprika, and curry powder for seasoning.
2. Coat the base of your Crock Pot with butter.
3. At first, make a layer of red potatoes in the cooker.
4. Now add layers of sweet potatoes and onion.
5. Add corns and tomatoes on top.
6. Whisk yogurt with baking soda, flour, and apple cider vinegar in a bowl.
7. Add the yogurt-flour mixture on top of the layers of veggies.
8. Lastly, drizzle the shredded cheese over it.
9. Put the cooker's lid on and set the cooking time to 6 hours on High settings.
10. Slice and serve.

**Nutrition Info:**
- Info Per Serving: Calories 272, Total Fat 1.9g, Fiber 4g, Total Carbs 51.34g, Protein 14g

## Cheddar Mushrooms

Servings:4 | Cooking Time: 6 Hours

**Ingredients:**
- 4 cups cremini mushrooms, sliced
- 1 teaspoon dried oregano
- 1 teaspoon ground black pepper
- ½ teaspoon salt
- 1 cup Cheddar cheese, shredded
- 1 cup heavy cream
- 1 cup of water

**Directions:**
1. Pour water and heavy cream in the Crock Pot.
2. Add salt, ground black pepper, and dried oregano.
3. Then add sliced mushrooms, and Cheddar cheese.
4. Cook the meal on Low for 6 hours.
5. When the mushrooms are cooked, gently stir them and transfer in the serving plates.

**Nutrition Info:**
- InfoPer Serving: 239 calories, 9.6g protein, 4.8g carbohydrates, 20.6g fat, 0.7g fiber, 71mg cholesterol, 484mg sodium, 386m potassium.

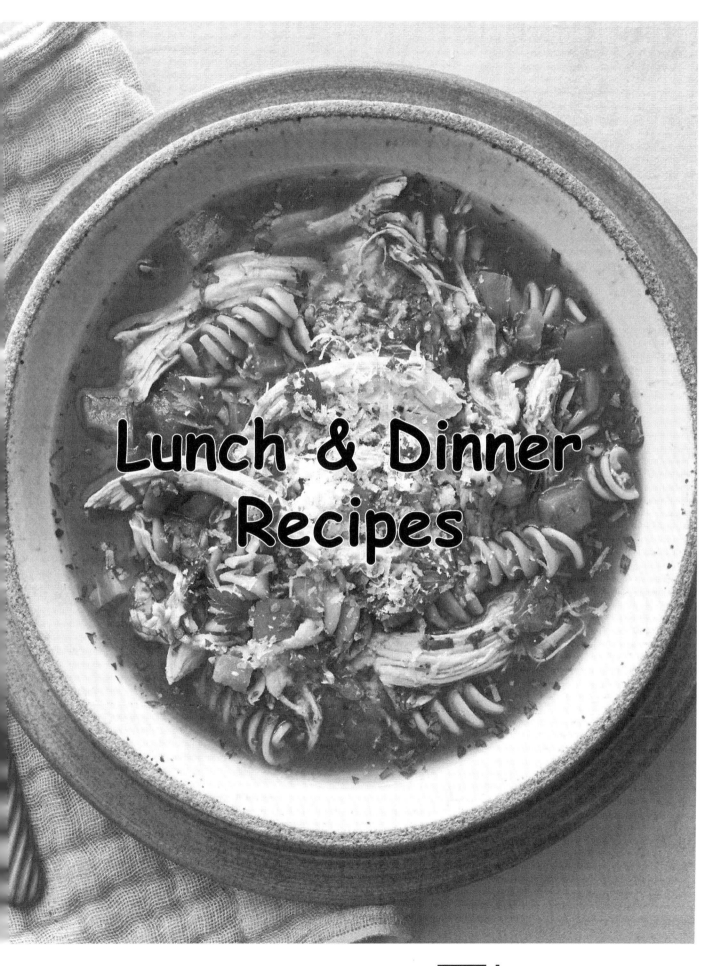

# Lunch & Dinner Recipes

# Lunch & Dinner Recipes

## Creamy Panade

Servings:4 | Cooking Time: 2.5 Hours

**Ingredients:**
- 5 oz bread, toasted, chopped
- 1 teaspoon garlic powder
- ½ cup red kidney beans, canned
- ¼ cup Mozzarella, shredded
- 3 cups of water
- 6 oz sausages, chopped

**Directions:**
1. Put chopped sausages in the Crock Pot.
2. Add water, cheese, red kidney beans, garlic powder, and bread.
3. Gently stir the mixture and close the lid.
4. Cook the panade on high for 2.5 hours.

**Nutrition Info:**
- InfoPer Serving: 323 calories,16.8g protein, 32.6g carbohydrates, 13.8g fat, 4.4g fiber, 37mg cholesterol, 579mg sodium 483mg potassium.

## Red Wine Vegetable Stew

Servings: 8 | Cooking Time: 6 1/2 Hours

**Ingredients:**
- 2 tablespoons olive oil
- 1 large onion, chopped
- 2 garlic cloves, minced
- 2 large carrots, sliced
- 2 parsnips, diced
- 2 sweet potatoes, peeled and cubed
- 2 red potatoes, peeled and cubed
- 1 cup diced tomatoes
- 4 Portobello mushrooms, sliced
- 1/2 cup red wine
- 1 1/2 cups vegetable stock
- 1 bay leaf
- 1 thyme sprig
- Salt and pepper to taste

**Directions:**
1. Heat the oil in a skillet and add the onion and garlic. Cook for 2 minutes until softened then transfer in your Crock Pot.
2. Add the remaining ingredients and season with salt and pepper.
3. Cook on low settings for 6 hours.
4. Serve the stew warm and fresh.

## Beans Chili

Servings: 2 | Cooking Time: 3 Hours

**Ingredients:**
- ½ red bell pepper, chopped
- ½ green bell pepper, chopped
- 1 garlic clove, minced
- ½ cup yellow onion, chopped
- ½ cup roasted tomatoes, crushed
- 1 cup canned red kidney beans, drained
- 1 cup canned white beans, drained
- 1 cup canned black beans, drained
- ½ cup corn
- Salt and black pepper to the taste
- 1 tablespoon chili powder
- 1 cup veggie stock

**Directions:**
1. In your Crock Pot, mix the peppers with the beans and the other ingredients, toss, put the lid on and cook on High for 3 hours.
2. Divide into bowls and serve right away.

**Nutrition Info:**
- Info calories 400, fat 14, fiber 5, carbs 29, protein 22

# Vegetarian Fajitas

Servings: 6 | Cooking Time: 6 1/4 Hours

**Ingredients:**

- 2 tablespoons olive oil
- 2 red bell peppers, cored and sliced
- 1 yellow bell pepper, cored and sliced
- 1 shallot, sliced
- 4 garlic cloves, chopped
- 1/4 teaspoon chili powder
- 1/4 teaspoon cumin powder
- 1 tablespoon soy sauce
- 12 oz. seitan, crumbled
- 1/2 cup vegetable stock
- 1/2 cup tomato sauce
- Salt and pepper to taste
- Flour tortillas for serving

**Directions:**

1. Heat the oil in a skillet and add the seitan. Cook until golden then transfer in your Crock Pot.
2. Add the remaining ingredients and season with salt and pepper.
3. Cook on low settings for 6 hours.
4. Serve the fajitas warm, wrapped in tortillas.

# Cuban Pork Chops

Servings: 6 | Cooking Time: 6 1/4 Hours

**Ingredients:**

6 pork chops
2 large onions, sliced
1 teaspoon grated ginger
1 teaspoon cumin seeds
4 garlic cloves, chopped
1 teaspoon chili powder
1 lemon, juiced
1 bay leaf
Salt and pepper to taste
1 cup chicken stock

**Directions:**

1. Mix all the ingredients in your Crock Pot, adjusting the taste with salt and pepper.
2. Cover and cook on low settings for 6 hours.
3. Serve the pork chops warm.

# Beef Okra Tomato Stew

Servings: 6 | Cooking Time: 6 1/4 Hours

**Ingredients:**

1 1/2 pounds beef roast, cut into thin strips
1 large onion, chopped
4 garlic cloves, minced
1 can (15 oz.) diced tomatoes
12 oz. frozen okra, chopped
2 large potatoes, peeled and cubed
1 cup beef stock
1 thyme sprig
Salt and pepper to taste
Chopped parsley for serving

**Directions:**

1. Combine the beef roast, onion, garlic, tomatoes, okra, potatoes, stock and thyme sprig in your crock pot.
2. Add salt and pepper to taste and cook on low settings for 6 hours.
3. Serve the stew warm and fresh or chilled, topped with chopped parsley.

# French Onion Roasted Pork Chop

Servings: 6 | Cooking Time: 6 1/4 Hours

**Ingredients:**
- 6 pork chops
- 1/4 cup white wine
- 1 can condensed onion soup
- 1 teaspoon garlic powder
- Salt and pepper to taste

**Directions:**
1. Combine all the ingredients in your Crock Pot.
2. Add salt and pepper to taste and cover with a lid.
3. Cook on low settings for 6 hours.
4. Serve the pork chops warm.

# Curried Beef Short Ribs

Servings: 6 | Cooking Time: 8 1/4 Hours

**Ingredients:**
- 4 pounds beef short ribs
- 3 tablespoons red curry paste
- 1 cup tomato sauce
- 1 teaspoon curry powder
- 1/2 teaspoon garlic powder
- 2 shallots, chopped
- 1 teaspoon grated ginger
- 1 lime, juiced
- Salt and pepper to taste

**Directions:**
1. Mix the curry paste, tomato sauce, curry powder, garlic powder, shallots, ginger and lime juice in a crock pot.
2. Add salt and pepper then place the ribs in the pot as well.
3. Coat the ribs well and cover with a lid. Cook on low settings for 8 hours.
4. Serve the ribs warm and fresh.

# Hearty Bbq Pork Belly

Servings: 8 | Cooking Time: 7 1/4 Hours

**Ingredients:**
- 4 pounds pork belly, trimmed
- 2 cups BBQ sauce
- 2 chipotle peppers, chopped
- 2 red onions, sliced
- 6 garlic cloves, chopped
- 1 teaspoon salt
- 1 thyme sprig

**Directions:**
1. Combine all the ingredients in your Crock Pot.
2. Cover and cook on low settings for 7 hours.
3. Serve the pork belly warm with your favorite side dish.

# Pork Roast And Olives

Servings: 2 | Cooking Time: 6 Hours

**Ingredients:**
- 1 pound pork roast, sliced
- ½ cup black olives, pitted and halved
- ½ cup kalamata olives, pitted and halved
- 2 medium carrots, chopped
- ½ cup tomato sauce
- 1 small yellow onion, chopped
- 2 garlic cloves, minced
- 1 bay leaf
- Salt and black pepper to the taste

**Directions:**
1. In your Crock Pot, mix the pork roast with the olives and the other ingredients, toss, put the lid on and cook on High for 6 hours.
2. Divide everything between plates and serve.

**Nutrition Info:**
Info calories 360, fat 4, fiber 3, carbs 17, protein 27

# Fennel Braised Chicken

Servings: 4 | Cooking Time: 6 1/4 Hours

**Ingredients:**
- 4 chicken breasts
- 1 fennel bulb, sliced
- 1 sweet onion, sliced
- 2 carrots, sliced
- 2 oranges, juiced
- 1 bay leaf
- 1 1/2 cups chicken stock
- Salt and pepper to taste

**Directions:**
1. Combine all the ingredients in your crock pot.
2. Add salt and pepper to taste and cook on low settings for 6 hours.
3. Serve the chicken warm.

# Thai Style Butternut Squash Tofu Stew

Servings: 6 | Cooking Time: 6 1/2 Hours

**Ingredients:**
- 8 oz. firm tofu, cubed
- 2 tablespoons olive oil
- 2 carrots, sliced
- 2 cups butternut squash cubes
- 1 pinch chili powder
- 1/2 teaspoon grated ginger
- 1 lemongrass stalk, crushed
- 1/4 teaspoon cumin seeds
- 1/2 teaspoon turmeric powder
- Salt and pepper to taste

**Directions:**
1. Heat the oil in a skillet and add the tofu. Cook on all sides until golden brown. Transfer in your Crock Pot and add the remaining ingredients.
2. Cook the stew on low settings for 6 hours.
3. The stew is best served warm.

## Seitan Chow Mein

Servings: 6 | Cooking Time: 2 1/4 Hours

**Ingredients:**
- 1/2 pound seitan, diced
- 2 celery stalks, sliced
- 2 carrots, sliced
- 2 green onions, chopped
- 2 tablespoons soy sauce
- 1/2 cup vegetable stock
- 1 pinch chili flakes
- 1 cup green peas
- 1 cup water chestnuts, chopped
- 1 tablespoon cornstarch
- 1/4 cup cold water

**Directions:**
1. Combine the seitan, celery, carrots, green onions, soy sauce, stock, chili flakes, green peas and water chestnuts in your crock pot.
2. Cook on high settings for 1 hour then add the cornstarch and water and cook for 1 additional hour.
3. Serve the dish warm and fresh.

## Lime Bean Stew

Servings: 8 | Cooking Time: 6 1/4 Hours

**Ingredients:**
- 2 cups dried lime beans
- 2 carrots, sliced
- 2 celery stalks, sliced
- 1 head cauliflower, cut into florets
- 1 teaspoon grated ginger
- 1 cup diced tomatoes
- 1 cup tomato sauce
- 2 cups vegetable stock
- 1 bay leaf
- 1 thyme sprig
- Salt and pepper to taste

**Directions:**
1. Combine the beans, carrots, celery, cauliflower, ginger, tomatoes, tomato sauce, stock, salt and pepper, as well as bay leaf and thyme in your crock pot.
2. Season with salt and pepper as needed and cook on low settings for 6 hours.
3. The stew is best served warm.

# Greek Style Chicken Ragout

Servings: 8 | Cooking Time: 8 1/4 Hours

**Ingredients:**
4 chicken breasts, halved
1 pound new potatoes, washed
1 pound baby carrots
1 zucchini, cubed
4 garlic cloves, chopped
1 sweet onion, sliced
4 artichoke hearts, chopped
1 lemon, juiced
1 teaspoon dried oregano
Salt and pepper to taste
1 1/2 cups chicken stock

**Directions:**
. Combine the chicken, potatoes, carrots, zucchini, garlic, onion, artichoke hearts, lemon juice, oregano and stock in your Crock Pot.
. Add salt and pepper to taste and cover with a lid.
. Cook on low settings for 8 hours.
. Serve the chicken and veggies warm.

# Lemon Vegetable Pork Roast

Servings: 8 | Cooking Time: 8 1/4 Hours

**Ingredients:**
1 large onion, sliced
4 pounds pork roast, cut into quarters
1/2 pounds baby carrots
2 cups snap peas
2 parsnips, sliced
2 large potatoes, peeled and cubed
1 cup vegetable stock
1 tablespoon molasses
1/4 cup red wine vinegar
2 tablespoons soy sauce
2 tablespoon ketchup
1 teaspoon garlic powder
1/4 teaspoon cayenne pepper
Salt and pepper to taste
1 lemon, sliced

**Directions:**
. Combine the onion, pork roast, baby carrots, snap peas, parsnips, potatoes, stock, molasses, vinegar, soy sauce, ketchup, garlic powder and cayenne pepper in your Crock Pot.
. Add salt and pepper to taste and cover with lemon slices. Cover the pot with its lid.
. Cook on low settings for 8 hours.
. Serve the roast warm and fresh.

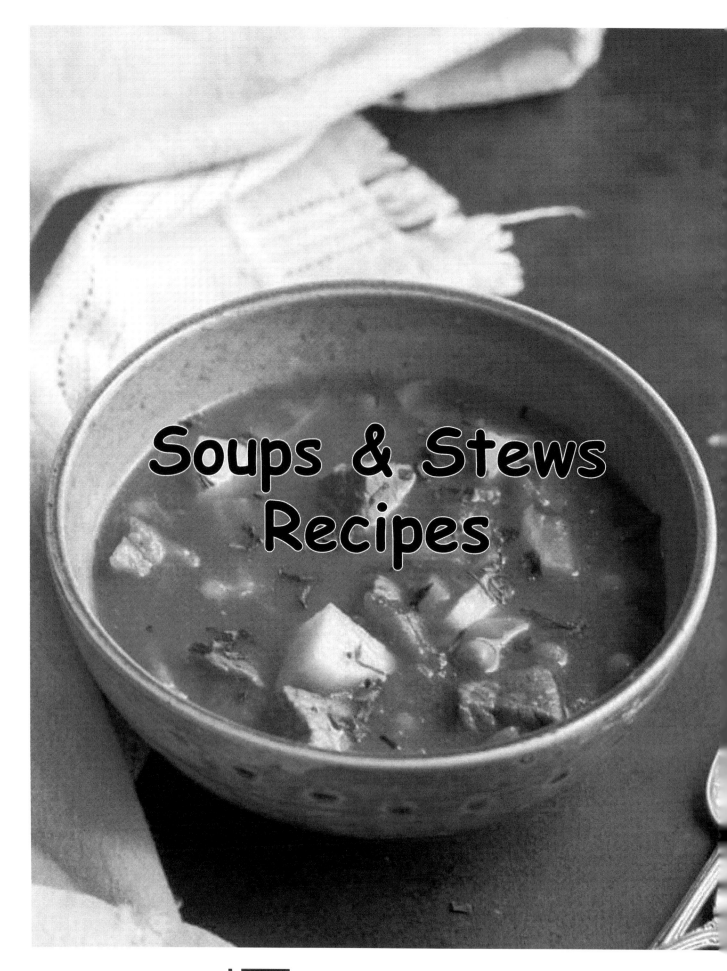

Soups & Stews
Recipes

# Soups & Stews Recipes

## Curried Vegetable Soup

Servings: 10 | Cooking Time: 6 1/2 Hours

**Ingredients:**
- 1 sweet onion, finely chopped
- 4 garlic cloves, chopped
- 2 tablespoons olive oil
- 1 teaspoon grated ginger
- 1/2 head cauliflower, cut into florets
- 2 large potatoes, peeled and cubed
- 1/2 head cabbage, shredded
- 2 tomatoes, peeled and diced
- 1 cup green peas
- 2 tablespoons red curry paste
- 2 cups vegetable stock
- 4 cups water
- 1/2 lemongrass talk, crushed
- Salt and pepper to taste

**Directions:**
1. Heat the olive oil in a skillet and stir in the onion and garlic. Cook for 2 minutes then add the ginger and curry paste. Sauté for 2 additional minutes then transfer in your Crock Pot.
2. Add the cauliflower, potatoes, cabbage, tomatoes, green peas, stock and water, as well as the lemongrass stalk.
3. Season with salt and pepper and cook on low settings for 6 hours.
4. Serve the soup warm.

## Curried Turkey Soup

Servings: 8 | Cooking Time: 6 1/2 Hours

**Ingredients:**
- 2 tablespoons olive oil
- 1 1/2 pounds turkey breast, cubed
- 2 carrots, diced
- 1 sweet onion, chopped
- 1 celery stalk, sliced
- 2 garlic cloves, chopped
- 1 teaspoon grated ginger
- 1 cup coconut milk
- 3 cups chicken stock
- 1 cup water
- 1 tablespoon curry powder
- Salt and pepper to taste

**Directions:**
1. Heat the oil in a skillet and stir in the turkey. Cook on all sides for a few minutes until golden then transfer in your Crock Pot.
2. Add the carrots, onion, celery, garlic, ginger, coconut milk, stock, water and curry powder.
3. Season with salt and pepper and cook on low settings for 6 hours.
4. Serve the soup warm.

# Tender Mushroom Stew

Servings:6 | Cooking Time: 8 Hours

**Ingredients:**
- 1-pound cremini mushrooms, chopped
- 1 cup carrot, grated
- 1 yellow onion, diced
- 2 teaspoons dried basil
- ½ cup greek yogurt
- ½ cup rutabaga, chopped
- 5 cups beef broth

**Directions:**
1. Put all ingredients in the Crock Pot.
2. Close the lid and cook the stew on Low for 8 hours.

**Nutrition Info:**
- InfoPer Serving: 84 calories, 8.1g protein, g carbohydrates, 1.6g fat, 1.6g fiber, 1mg cholesterol, 662mg sodium, 660mg potassium

# Taco Spices Stew

Servings:4 | Cooking Time: 8 Hours

**Ingredients:**
- 1-pound beef sirloin
- 1 teaspoon liquid honey
- 3 cups of water
- 1 cup sweet potato, chopped
- 1 teaspoon salt
- 1 teaspoon taco seasonings

**Directions:**
1. Cut the beef sirloin into the strips and sprinkle with taco seasonings.
2. Then transfer the beef strips in the Crock Pot.
3. Add salt, sweet potato, water, and liquid honey.
4. Close the lid and cook the stew for 8 hours on Low.

**Nutrition Info:**
- InfoPer Serving: 264 calories, 35.4g protein, 12.3g carbohydrates, 7.2g fat, 1.7g fiber, 101mg cholesterol, 732mg sodium, 697mg potassium.

# Lentil Stew

Servings:4 | Cooking Time: 6 Hours

**Ingredients:**
- 2 cups chicken stock
- ½ cup red lentils
- 1 eggplant, chopped
- 1 tablespoon tomato paste
- 1 cup of water
- 1 teaspoon Italian seasonings

**Directions:**
1. Mix chicken stock with red lentils and tomato paste.
2. Pour the mixture in the Crock Pot.
3. Add eggplants and Italian seasonings.
4. Cook the stew on low for 6 hours.

**Nutrition Info:**
- InfoPer Serving: 125 calories, 7.8g protein, 22.4g carbohydrates, 1.1g fat, 11.5g fiber, 1mg cholesterol, 392mg sodium, 540mg potassium.

## Summer Vegetable Soup

Servings: 8 | Cooking Time: 6 1/2 Hours

**Ingredients:**

- 1 sweet onion, chopped
- 1 garlic clove, chopped
- 2 tablespoons olive oil
- 1 zucchini, cubed
- 1 yellow squash, cubed
- 1/2 head cauliflower, cut into florets
- 1/2 head broccoli, cut into florets
- 2 ripe tomatoes, peeled and cubed
- 1 carrot, sliced
- 1 celery stalk, sliced
- 1/2 cup edamame
- 2 cups chicken stock
- 5 cups water
- Salt and pepper to taste
- 1 lemon, juiced
- 1 tablespoon chopped parsley

**Directions:**

1. Combine the onion, garlic, olive oil and the rest of the ingredients in your Crock Pot.
2. Add salt and pepper to taste and cook on low settings for 6 hours.
3. When done, stir in the lemon juice and parsley and serve the soup warm or chilled.

## Stuffed Bell Pepper Soup

Servings: 6 | Cooking Time: 8 1/2 Hours

**Ingredients:**

- 6 medium size red bell peppers, cored
- 1 pound ground pork
- 1/2 pound ground beef
- 2 shallots, chopped
- 1 carrot, grated
- 1/4 cup white rice
- 2 tablespoons chopped parsley
- 1 teaspoon dried thyme
- 1/4 teaspoon cumin powder
- Salt and pepper to taste
- 2 cups beef stock
- 6 cups water
- 1 can fire roasted tomatoes
- 1 bay leaf
- 1 thyme sprig
- 1 lemon, juiced

**Directions:**

1. In a bowl, mix the ground pork, beef, shallots, carrot, rice, chopped parsley, thyme and cumin powder. Add salt and pepper to taste and mix well.
2. Stuff each bell pepper with the meat mixture and place them all in your Crock Pot.
3. Add the remaining ingredients and season with salt and pepper.
4. Cook on low settings for 8 hours.
5. Serve the soup warm.

## Okra Vegetable Soup

Servings: 8 | Cooking Time: 7 1/4 Hours

**Ingredients:**

- 1 pound ground beef
- 2 tablespoons canola oil
- 2 shallots, chopped
- 1 carrot, sliced
- 1 can fire roasted tomatoes, chopped
- 2 cups chopped okra
- 1/2 cup green peas
- 2 potatoes, peeled and cubed
- 1/2 cup sweet corn, drained
- Salt and pepper to taste
- 2 cups water
- 2 cups chicken stock
- 1 lemon, juiced

**Directions:**

1. Heat the oil in a skillet and stir in the beef. Cook for a few minutes then transfer the meat in your Crock Pot.
2. Add the shallots, carrot, tomatoes, okra, peas, potatoes, corn, water and stock, as well as lemon juice, salt and pepper.
3. Cook the soup on low settings for 7 hours.
4. Serve the soup warm and fresh.

# Hot And Sour Soup

Servings: 8 | Cooking Time: 7 1/2 Hours

**Ingredients:**
- 2 oz. dried shiitake mushrooms
- 1 pound fresh mushrooms, sliced
- 1 can (8 oz.) bamboo shoots, drained
- 2 carrots, sliced
- 1 sweet onion, chopped
- 14 oz. tofu, cubed
- 1/2 head green cabbage, shredded
- 1 teaspoon grated ginger
- 1/2 teaspoon chili flakes
- 2 cups chicken stock
- 5 cups water
- 2 tablespoons soy sauce
- 2 tablespoons rice vinegar
- 2 green onions, sliced

**Directions:**
1. Place the shiitake mushrooms in a bowl and cover them with boiling water. Allow to rehydrate for 10 minutes then chop and place in your Crock Pot.
2. Add the remaining ingredients, except the green onions and cook on low settings for 7 hours.
3. When done, stir in the green onions and serve right away.

# Beef Mushroom Soup

Servings: 8 | Cooking Time: 8 1/2 Hours

**Ingredients:**
- 1 pound beef roast, cubed
- 2 tablespoons canola oil
- 1 sweet onion, chopped
- 2 garlic cloves, chopped
- 1 pound mushrooms, sliced
- 1 can fire roasted tomatoes
- 2 cups beef stock
- 5 cups water
- 1 bay leaf
- 1 thyme sprig
- 1/2 teaspoon caraway seeds
- Salt and pepper to taste

**Directions:**
1. Heat the oil in a skillet and stir in the beef roast. Cook on all sides for a few minutes then transfer in your Crock Pot.
2. Add the onion, garlic, mushrooms, tomatoes, stock and water, as well as bay leaf and thyme sprig, plus the caraway seeds.
3. Season with salt and pepper and cook on low settings for 8 hours.
4. The soup is best served warm.

# Mixed Bean Vegetarian Soup

Servings: 8 | Cooking Time: 4 1/4 Hours

**Ingredients:**
- 1 tablespoon olive oil
- 1 sweet onion, chopped
- 1 garlic clove, chopped
- 1 carrot, diced
- 1 celery stalk, sliced
- 1 red bell pepper, cored and diced
- 1/2 teaspoon chili powder
- 1/2 teaspoon cumin powder
- 2 cups vegetable stock
- 1 can (15 oz.) white bean, drained
- 1 can (15 oz.) cannellini beans, drained
- 1 cup diced tomatoes
- 2 cups water
- Salt and pepper to taste
- 2 tablespoons chopped cilantro
- 1 lime, juiced
- 1 avocado, peeled and sliced

**Directions:**
1. Heat the oil in a skillet and add the onion, carrot, garlic and celery. Cook for 5 minutes until softened.
2. Transfer in your Crock Pot and stir in the remaining ingredients, except the cilantro, lime and avocado.
3. Adjust the taste with salt and pepper and cook on low settings for 4 hours.
4. When done, pour the soup into serving bowls and top with cilantro and avocado.
5. Drizzle with lime juice and serve right away.

# Ham And Sweet Potato Soup

Servings: 6 | Cooking Time: 3 1/2 Hours

**Ingredients:**
- 1 1/2 cups diced ham
- 1 sweet onion, chopped
- 1 carrot, diced
- 1 celery stalk, diced
- 1 parsnip, diced
- 2 large sweet potatoes, peeled and cubed
- 2 cups chicken stock
- 2 cups water
- 1 bay leaf
- 1 thyme sprig
- Salt and pepper to taste

**Directions:**
1. Combine all the ingredients in your Crock Pot.
2. Add salt and pepper to taste and cook on high settings for 3 hours.
3. Serve the soup warm and fresh.

# Lobster Soup

Servings:4 | Cooking Time: 2 Hours

**Ingredients:**
- 4 cups of water
- 1-pound lobster tail, chopped
- ½ cup fresh cilantro, chopped
- 1 cup coconut cream
- 1 teaspoon ground coriander
- 1 garlic clove, diced

**Directions:**
1. Pour water and coconut cream in the Crock Pot.
2. Add a lobster tail, cilantro, and ground coriander.
3. Then add the garlic clove and close the lid.
4. Cook the lobster soup on High for 2 hours.

**Nutrition Info:**
- InfoPer Serving: 241 calories, 23g protein, 3.6g carbohydrates, 15.2g fat, 1.4g fiber, 165mg cholesterol, 568mg sodium, 435mg potassium.

# Chicken Chickpea Soup

Servings: 6 | Cooking Time: 6 1/2 Hours

**Ingredients:**
- 2 chicken breasts, cubed
- 2 tablespoons olive oil
- 2 shallots, chopped
- 1 pound potatoes, peeled and diced
- 1 can (15 oz.) chickpeas, drained
- 2 cups chicken stock
- 4 cups water
- 2 tablespoons lemon juice
- 1 teaspoon dried tarragon
- Salt and pepper to taste
- 1 cup buttermilk

**Directions:**
1. Heat the oil in a skillet and add the chicken. Cook on all sides until golden then transfer in your Crock Pot.
2. Add the remaining ingredients, except the buttermilk, and cook on low settings for 6 hours.
3. When done, add the buttermilk and serve the soup warm.

# Coconut Cod Stew

Servings:6 | Cooking Time: 6.5 Hours

**Ingredients:**
- 1-pound cod fillet, chopped
- 2 oz scallions, roughly chopped
- 1 cup coconut cream
- 1 teaspoon curry powder
- 1 teaspoon garlic, diced

**Directions:**
1. Mix curry powder with coconut cream and garlic.
2. Add scallions and gently stir the liquid.
3. After this, pour it in the Crock Pot and add cod fillet.
4. Stir the stew mixture gently and close the lid.
5. Cook the stew on low for 6.5 hours.

**Nutrition Info:**
- InfoPer Serving: 158 calories, 14.7g protein, 3.3g carbohydrates, 10.3g fat, 1.3g fiber, 37mg cholesterol, 55mg sodium, 138mg potassium.

# Tomato Beef Soup

Servings: 8 | Cooking Time: 8 1/4 Hours

**Ingredients:**
- 2 tablespoons olive oil
- 2 bacon slices, chopped
- 2 pounds beef roast, cubed
- 2 sweet onions, chopped
- 2 tomatoes, peeled and diced
- 2 cups tomato sauce
- 1 cup beef stock
- 3 cups water
- Salt and pepper to taste
- 1 thyme sprig
- 1 rosemary sprig

**Directions:**
1. Heat the oil in a skillet and add the bacon. Cook until crisp and stir in the beef roast. Cook for 5 minutes on all sides.
2. Transfer the beet and bacon in a Crock Pot.
3. Add the remaining ingredients and adjust the taste with salt and pepper.
4. Cook on low settings for 8 hours.
5. Serve the soup warm or chilled.

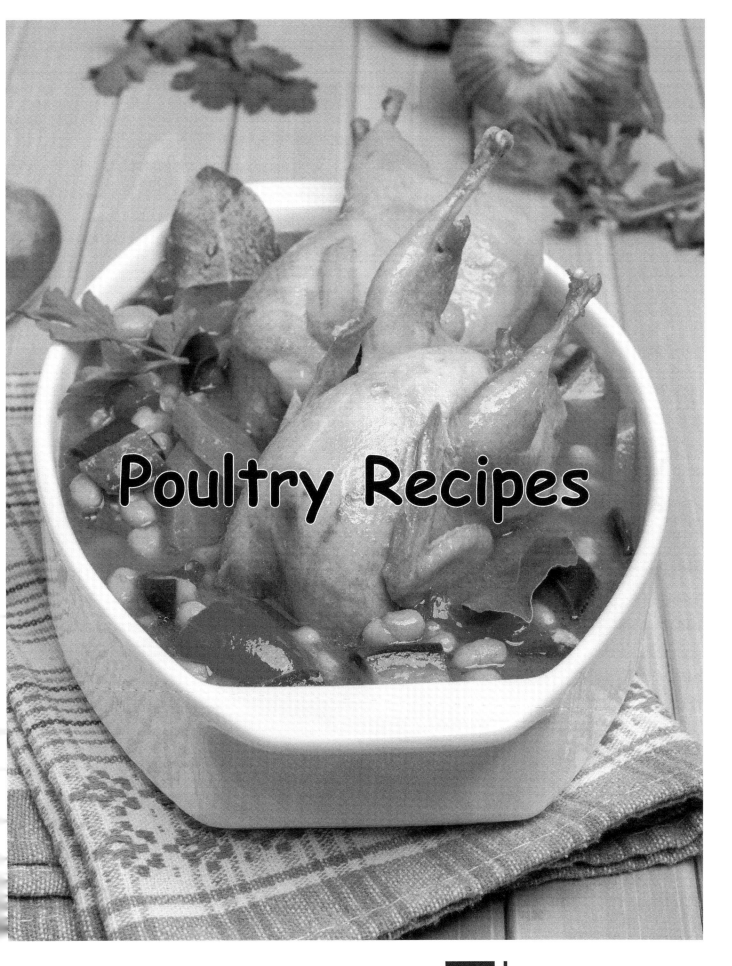

Poultry Recipes

# Poultry Recipes

## Crockpot Chicken Curry

Servings:6 | Cooking Time: 8 Hours

**Ingredients:**
- 2 pounds chicken breasts, bones removed
- 1 can coconut milk
- 1 onion, chopped
- 4 tablespoons curry powder
- Salt and pepper to taste

**Directions:**
1. Place all ingredients in the crockpot.
2. Give a good stir to incorporate everything.
3. Close the lid and cook on low for 8 hours or 6 hours on high.

**Nutrition Info:**
- Info Calories per serving:468; Carbohydrates: 9g; Protein: 34.5g; Fat: 33.7g; Sugar: 1.2g; Sodium:646 mg; Fiber: 1.6g

## Latin Chicken

Servings: 6 | Cooking Time: 5 Hours

**Ingredients:**
- 6 oz. sweet pepper, julienned
- 1 tsp salt
- 1 tsp chili flakes
- 21 oz. chicken thighs
- 1 onion, cut into petals
- 1 tsp garlic powder
- ½ cup salsa verde
- ¼ cup sweet corn, frozen
- 2 cups of water
- 1 peach, pitted, chopped
- 1 tsp canola oil

**Directions:**
1. Add chicken, salsa verde, and all other ingredients to the Crock Pot.
2. Put the cooker's lid on and set the cooking time to 5 hours on High settings.
3. Serve warm.

**Nutrition Info:**
- Info Per Serving: Calories: 182, Total Fat: 9.2g, Fiber: 1g, Total Carbs: 7.35g, Protein: 18g

## Chives Chicken Wings

Servings: 2 | Cooking Time: 6 Hours

**Ingredients:**
- 1 cup chicken stock
- 1 pound chicken wings
- ½ cup chives, chopped
- ½ teaspoon chili powder
- ½ teaspoon coriander, ground
- ½ teaspoon cumin, ground
- 1 teaspoon oregano, dried
- A pinch of salt and black pepper

**Directions:**
1. In your Crock Pot, mix the chicken with the stock, chives and the other ingredients, toss, put the lid on and cook on Low for 6 hours.
2. Divide the mix between plates and serve with a side salad.

**Nutrition Info:**
- Info calories 220, fat 8, fiber 2, carbs 5, protein 11

# Chicken Mix

Servings:4 | Cooking Time: 8 Hours

**Ingredients:**
- 1 cup carrot, chopped
- 1-pound chicken wings
- 1 cup of water
- ½ cup tomato juice
- 1 teaspoon salt
- 1 teaspoon dried rosemary

**Directions:**
1. Put chicken wings in the Crock Pot.
2. Add carrot, tomato juice, water, salt, and dried rosemary.
3. Close the lid and cook the meal on low for 8 hours.

**Nutrition Info:**
- InfoPer Serving: 233 calories, 33.3g protein, 4.2g carbohydrates, 8.g 5fat, 0.9g fiber, 101mg cholesterol, 781mg sodium, 437mg potassium.

# Garlic Turkey

Servings: 2 | Cooking Time: 6 Hours

**Ingredients:**
- 1 pound turkey breast, skinless, boneless and cubed
- 1 tablespoon avocado oil
- ½ cup chicken stock
- 2 tablespoons tomato paste
- 2 tablespoons garlic, minced
- ½ teaspoon chili powder
- ½ teaspoon oregano, dried
- A pinch of salt and black pepper
- 1 tablespoon parsley, chopped

**Directions:**
1. In your Crock Pot, mix the turkey with the oil, stock, tomato paste and the other ingredients, toss, put the lid on and cook on Low for 6 hours.
2. Divide the mix between plates and serve with a side salad.

**Nutrition Info:**
- Info calories 231, fat 7, fiber 2, carbs 6, protein 12

# Turkey Soup

Servings: 4 | Cooking Time: 3 Hours

**Ingredients:**
- 3 celery stalks, chopped
- 1 yellow onion, chopped
- 1 tablespoon olive oil
- 6 cups turkey stock
- Salt and black pepper to the taste
- ¼ cup parsley, chopped
- 3 cups baked spaghetti squash, chopped
- 3 cups turkey, cooked and shredded

**Directions:**
1. In your Crock Pot, mix oil with celery, onion, stock, salt, pepper, squash, turkey and parsley, stir, cover, cook on High for 3 hours, ladle into bowls and serve.

**Nutrition Info:**
- Info calories 250, fat 4, fiber 1, carbs 13, protein 10

# Chicken Broccoli Casserole

Servings: 4 | Cooking Time: 4 Hrs

**Ingredients:**
- 3 cups cheddar cheese, grated
- 10 oz. broccoli florets
- 3 chicken breasts, skinless, boneless, cooked and cubed
- 1 cup mayonnaise
- 1 tbsp olive oil
- 1/3 cup chicken stock
- Salt and black pepper to the taste
- Juice of 1 lemon

**Directions:**
1. Grease the base of your Crock Pot with olive oil.
2. Add chicken pieces, broccoli florets, and half of the cheese to the cooker.
3. Mix salt, lemon juice, black pepper, and mayo in a bowl.
4. Spread this lemon mixture over the chicken pieces and add the remaining cheese on top.
5. Put the cooker's lid on and set the cooking time to 4 hours on High settings.
6. Serve.

**Nutrition Info:**
- Info Per Serving: Calories: 320, Total Fat: 5g, Fiber: 4g, Total Carbs: 16g, Protein: 25g

# Algerian Chicken

Servings:2 | Cooking Time: 4 Hours

**Ingredients:**
- 6 oz chicken breast, skinless, boneless, sliced
- 1 teaspoon peanut oil
- 1 teaspoon harissa
- 1 teaspoon tomato paste
- 1 tablespoon sesame oil
- 1 cup tomatoes, canned
- ¼ cup of water

**Directions:**
1. Mix tomato paste with harissa, peanut oil, and sesame oil. Whisk the mixture and mix it with sliced chicken breast.
2. After this, transfer the chicken in the Crock Pot in one layer.
3. Add water and close the lid.
4. Cook the chicken on High for 4 hours.

**Nutrition Info:**
- InfoPer Serving: 204 calories, 19.1 protein, 5g carbohydrates, 11.8g fat, 1.2g fiber, 55mg cholesterol, 81mg sodium, 555mg potassium.

# Turkey Curry

Servings: 4 | Cooking Time: 4 Hours

**Ingredients:**
- 18 ounces turkey meat, minced
- 3 ounces spinach
- 20 ounces canned tomatoes, chopped
- 2 tablespoons coconut oil
- 2 tablespoons coconut cream
- 2 garlic cloves, minced
- 2 yellow onions, sliced
- 1 tablespoon coriander, ground
- 2 tablespoons ginger, grated
- 1 tablespoons turmeric powder
- 1 tablespoon cumin, ground
- Salt and black pepper to the taste
- 2 tablespoons chili powder

**Directions:**
1. In your Crock Pot, mix turkey with spinach, tomatoes, oil, cream, garlic, onion, coriander, ginger, turmeric, cumin, chili, salt and pepper, stir, cover and cook on High for 4 hours.
2. Divide into bowls and serve.

**Nutrition Info:**
- Info calories 240, fat 4, fiber 3, carbs 13, protein 12

# Chicken Bowl

Servings:6 | Cooking Time: 4 Hours

**Ingredients:**
- 1-pound chicken breast, skinless, boneless, chopped
- 1 cup sweet corn, frozen
- 1 teaspoon ground paprika
- 1 teaspoon onion powder
- 1 cup tomatoes, chopped
- 1 cup of water
- 1 teaspoon olive oil

**Directions:**
1. Mix chopped chicken breast with ground paprika and onion powder. Transfer it in the Crock Pot.
2. Add water and sweet corn. Cook the mixture on High for 4 hours.
3. Then drain the liquid and transfer the mixture in the bowl.
4. Add tomatoes and olive oil. Mix the meal.

**Nutrition Info:**
- InfoPer Serving: 122 calories, 17.2g protein, 6.3g carbohydrates, 3g fat, 1.1g fiber, 48mg cholesterol, 45mg sodium, 424mg potassium.

# Braised Chicken With Bay Leaf

Servings:4 | Cooking Time: 8 Hours

**Ingredients:**
- 1-pound chicken breast, skinless
- 1 teaspoon salt
- 4 bay leaves
- 1 teaspoon garlic powder
- 3 cups of water

**Directions:**
1. Put all ingredients in the Crock Pot and close the lid.
2. Cook the chicken on low for 8 hours.
3. Then chop the chicken and transfer in the bowls.
4. Add chicken liquid from the Crock Pot.

**Nutrition Info:**
- InfoPer Serving: 135 calories, 24.2g protein, 1.3g carbohydrates, 2.9g fat, 0.3g fiber, 73mg cholesterol, 645mg sodium, 434mg potassium.

# Coca Cola Chicken

Servings: 4 | Cooking Time: 4 Hours

**Ingredients:**
- 1 yellow onion, minced
- 4 chicken drumsticks
- 1 tablespoon balsamic vinegar
- 1 chili pepper, chopped
- 15 ounces coca cola
- Salt and black pepper to the taste
- 2 tablespoons olive oil

**Directions:**
1. Heat up a pan with the oil over medium-high heat, add chicken pieces, stir and brown them on all sides and then transfer them to your Crock Pot.
2. Add vinegar, chili, coca cola, salt and pepper, cover and cook on High for 4 hours.
3. Divide chicken mix between plates and serve.

**Nutrition Info:**
- Info calories 372, fat 14, fiber 3, carbs 20, protein 15

# Parsley Chicken Mix

Servings: 2 | Cooking Time: 5 Hours

**Ingredients:**
- 1 pound chicken breast, skinless, boneless and sliced
- ½ cup parsley, chopped
- 2 tablespoons olive oil
- 1 tablespoon pine nuts
- 1 tablespoon lemon juice
- ½ cup chicken stock
- ¼ cup black olives, pitted and halved
- 1 teaspoon hot paprika
- A pinch of salt and black pepper

**Directions:**
1. In a blender, mix the parsley with the oil, pine nuts and lemon juice and pulse well.
2. In your Crock Pot, mix the chicken with the parsley mix and the remaining ingredients, toss, put the lid on and cook on High for 5 hours.
3. Divide everything between plates and serve.

**Nutrition Info:**
- Info calories 263, fat 14, fiber 3, carbs 7, protein 16

# Coconut Turkey

Servings: 2 | Cooking Time: 5 Hours

**Ingredients:**
- 1 yellow onion, chopped
- 1 tablespoon olive oil
- 1 cup coconut cream
- ½ teaspoon curry powder
- 1 pound turkey breast, skinless, boneless and cubed
- 1 teaspoon turmeric powder
- ½ cup chicken stock
- 1 tablespoon parsley, chopped
- A pinch of salt and black pepper

**Directions:**
1. In your Crock Pot, mix the turkey with the onion, oil and the other ingredients except the cream and the parsley, stir, put the lid on and cook on High for 4 hours and 30 minutes.
2. Add the remaining ingredients, toss, put the lid on again, cook on High for 30 minutes more, divide the mix between plates and serve.

**Nutrition Info:**
- Info calories 283, fat 11, fiber 2, carbs 8, protein 15

# Cuban Chicken

Servings: 4 | Cooking Time: 4 Hours

**Ingredients:**
- 4 gold potatoes, cut into medium chunks
- 1 yellow onion, thinly sliced
- 4 big tomatoes, cut into medium chunks
- 1 chicken, cut into 8 pieces
- Salt and black pepper to the taste
- 2 bay leaves
- Salt and black pepper to the taste

**Directions:**
1. In your instant Crock Pot, mix potatoes with onion, chicken, tomato, bay leaves, salt and pepper, stir well, cover and cook on High for 4 hours.
2. Add more salt and pepper, discard bay leaves, divide chicken mix between plates and serve.

**Nutrition Info:**
- Info calories 263, fat 2, fiber 1, carbs 27, protein 14

# Butterychicken Wings

Servings: 6 | Cooking Time: 5 Hours

**Ingredients:**
- 14 oz. chicken wings
- 1 tsp onion powder
- 1 tsp chili flakes
- 1 tsp garlic powder
- 1 tsp cilantro
- 1 tsp olive oil
- 1/3 cup butter, melted
- 1 tbsp flour
- ¼ cup milk
- 1 tsp salt
- 1 tbsp heavy cream
- 1 egg, beaten

**Directions:**
1. Add chicken wings, butter, onion powder, salt, garlic powder, cilantro, olive oil, and chili flakes to the Crock Pot.
2. Mix well to coat the chicken wings with the spices.
3. Put the cooker's lid on and set the cooking time to 2 hours on High settings.
4. Beat egg with olive oil, milk, flour, and cream in a mixer.
5. Pour this cream mixture over the cooked chicken.
6. Put the cooker's lid on and set the cooking time to 3 hours on Low settings.
7. Serve warm.

**Nutrition Info:**
- Info Per Serving: Calories: 225, Total Fat: 16.2g, Fiber: 0g, Total Carbs: 2.64g, Protein: 17g

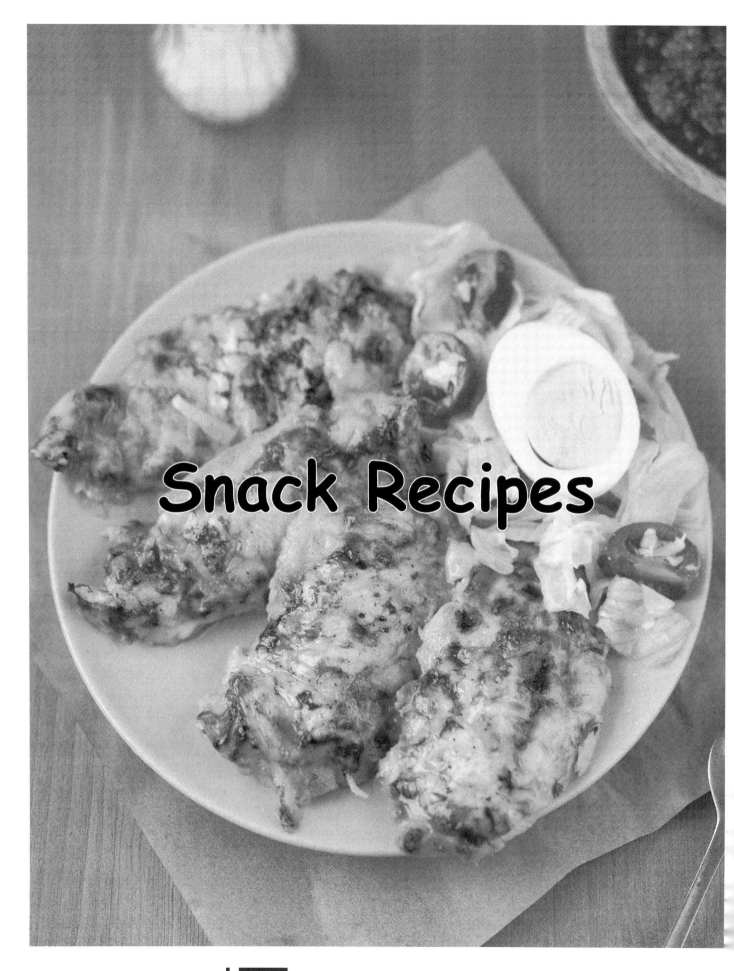

# Snack Recipes

# Snack Recipes

## Cheesy Pork Rolls

Servings: 8 | Cooking Time: 7 Hours

**Ingredients:**
- 3 oz. Monterey cheese, sliced
- 6 oz. ground pork
- 2 oz. onion, chopped
- 1 tbsp sliced garlic
- 1 tsp salt
- 1 tsp ground pepper
- 5 oz. Cheddar cheese, sliced
- 1 tbsp pesto sauce
- 8 flour tortilla
- 1 tsp olive oil

**Directions:**
1. Grease the base of your Crock Pot with olive oil.
2. Add ground pepper with onion, pesto sauce, ground pork, and onion to the Crock Pot.
3. Put the cooker's lid on and set the cooking time to 5 hours on High settings.
4. Mix well, then divide this beef mixture into each tortilla.
5. Drizzle chopped cheese over the tortilla filling.
6. Roll all the tortilla and place them in the Crock Pot.
7. Put the cooker's lid on and set the cooking time to 2 hours on High settings.
8. Serve.

**Nutrition Info:**
- Info Per Serving: Calories: 270, Total Fat: 10.8g, Fiber: 1g, Total Carbs: 27.52g, Protein: 16g

## Caramel Dip

Servings: 4 | Cooking Time: 2 Hours

**Ingredients:**
- 1 cup butter
- 12 ounces condensed milk
- 2 cups brown sugar
- 1 cup corn syrup

**Directions:**
1. In your Crock Pot, mix butter with condensed milk, sugar and corn syrup, cover and cook on High for 2 hours stirring often.
2. Divide into bowls and serve.

**Nutrition Info:**
- Info calories 172, fat 2, fiber 6, carbs 12, protein 4

## Chickpeas Spread

Servings: 2 | Cooking Time: 8 Hours

**Ingredients:**
- ½ cup chickpeas, dried
- 1 tablespoons olive oil
- 1 tablespoon lemon juice
- 1 cup veggie stock
- 1 tablespoon tahini
- A pinch of salt and black pepper
- 1 garlic clove, minced
- ½ tablespoon chives, chopped

**Directions:**
1. In your Crock Pot, combine the chickpeas with the stock, salt, pepper and the garlic, stir, put the lid on and cook on Low for 8 hours.
2. Drain chickpeas, transfer them to a blender, add the rest of the ingredients, pulse well, divide into bowls and serve as a party spread.

**Nutrition Info:**
- Info calories 211, fat 6, fiber 7, carbs 8, protein 4

# Bourbon Sausage Bites

Servings: 12 | Cooking Time: 3 Hours And 5 Minutes

**Ingredients:**
- 1/3 cup bourbon
- 1 pound smoked sausage, sliced
- 12 ounces chili sauce
- ¼ cup brown sugar
- 2 tablespoons yellow onion, grated

**Directions:**
1. Heat up a pan over medium-high heat, add sausage slices, brown them for 2 minutes on each side, drain them on paper towels and transfer to your Crock Pot.
2. Add chili sauce, sugar, onion and bourbon, toss to coat, cover and cook on Low for 3 hours.
3. Divide into bowls and serve as a snack.

**Nutrition Info:**
- Info calories 190, fat 11, fiber 1, carbs 12, protein 5

# Broccoli Dip

Servings: 2 | Cooking Time: 2 Hours

**Ingredients:**
- 1 green chili pepper, minced
- 2 tablespoons heavy cream
- 1 cup broccoli florets
- 1 tablespoon mayonnaise
- 2 tablespoons cream cheese, cubed
- A pinch of salt and black pepper
- 1 tablespoon chives, chopped

**Directions:**
1. In your Crock Pot, mix the broccoli with the chili pepper, mayo and the other ingredients, toss, put the lid on and cook on Low for 2 hours.
2. Blend using an immersion blender, divide into bowls and serve as a party dip.

**Nutrition Info:**
- Info calories 202, fat 3, fiber 3, carbs 7, protein 6

# Eggplant Zucchini Dip

Servings: 4 | Cooking Time: 4 Hrs 10 Minutes

**Ingredients:**
- 1 eggplant
- 1 zucchini, chopped
- 2 tbsp olive oil
- 2 tbsp balsamic vinegar
- 1 tbsp parsley, chopped
- 1 yellow onion, chopped
- 1 celery stick, chopped
- 1 tomato, chopped
- 2 tbsp tomato paste
- 1 and ½ tsp garlic, minced
- A pinch of sea salt
- Black pepper to the taste

**Directions:**
1. Rub the eggplant with cooking oil and grill it for 5 minutes per side on a preheated grill.
2. Chop the grilled eggplant and transfer it to the Crock Pot.
3. Add tomato, parsley and all other ingredients to the cooker.
4. Put the cooker's lid on and set the cooking time to 4 hours on High settings.
5. Serve.

**Nutrition Info:**
- Info Per Serving: Calories: 110, Total Fat: 1g, Fiber: 2g, Total Carbs: 7g, Protein: 5g

## Salmon Bites

Servings: 2 | Cooking Time: 2 Hours

**Ingredients:**
- 1 pound salmon fillets, boneless
- ¼ cup chili sauce
- A pinch of salt and black pepper
- ½ teaspoon turmeric powder
- 2 tablespoons grape jelly

**Directions:**
1. In your Crock Pot, mix the salmon with the chili sauce and the other ingredients, toss gently, put the lid on and cook on High for 2 hours.
2. Serve as an appetizer.

**Nutrition Info:**
- Info calories 200, fat 6, fiber 3, carbs 15, protein 12

## Tostadas

Servings: 4 | Cooking Time: 4 Hours

**Ingredients:**
- 4 pounds pork shoulder, boneless and cubed
- Salt and black pepper to the taste
- 2 cups coca cola
- 1/3 cup brown sugar
- ½ cup hot sauce
- 2 teaspoons chili powder
- 2 tablespoons tomato paste
- ¼ teaspoon cumin, ground
- 1 cup enchilada sauce
- Corn tortillas, toasted for a few minutes in the oven
- Mexican cheese, shredded for serving
- 4 shredded lettuce leaves, for serving
- Salsa
- Guacamole for serving

**Directions:**
1. In your Crock Pot, mix 1 cup coke with hot sauce, salsa, sugar, tomato paste, chili powder, cumin and pork, stir, cover and cook on Low for 4 hours.
2. Drain juice from the Crock Pot, transfer meat to a cutting board, shred it, return it to Crock Pot, add the rest of the coke and enchilada sauce and stir.
3. Place tortillas on a working surface, divide pork mix, lettuce leaves, Mexican cheese and guacamole and serve as a snack.

**Nutrition Info:**
- Info calories 162, fat 3, fiber 6, carbs 12, protein 5

## Blue Cheese Parsley Dip

Servings: 7 | Cooking Time: 7 Hours

**Ingredients:**
- 1 cup parsley, chopped
- 8 oz. celery stalk, chopped
- 6 oz. Blue cheese, chopped
- 1 tbsp apple cider vinegar
- 6 oz. cream
- 1 tsp minced garlic
- 1 tsp paprika
- ¼ tsp ground red pepper
- 1 onion, peeled and grated

**Directions:**
1. Whisk the cream with cream cheese in a bowl and add to the Crock Pot.
2. Toss in parsley, celery stalk, garlic, onion, apple cider vinegar, and red pepper ground.
3. Put the cooker's lid on and set the cooking time to 7 hours on Low settings.
4. Mix the dip after 4 hours of cooking then resume cooked.
5. Serve.

**Nutrition Info:**
- Info Per Serving: Calories: 151, Total Fat: 11.9g, Fiber: 1g, Total Carbs: 5.14g, Protein: 7g

# Herbed Pecans Snack

Servings: 5 | Cooking Time: 2 Hrs 15 Minutes

**Ingredients:**
- 1 lb. pecans halved
- 2 tbsp olive oil
- 1 tsp basil, dried
- 1 tbsp chili powder
- 1 tsp oregano, dried
- ¼ tsp garlic powder
- 1 tsp thyme, dried
- ½ tsp onion powder
- A pinch of cayenne pepper

**Directions:**
1. Add pecans, basil, and all other ingredients to the Crock Pot.
2. Put the cooker's lid on and set the cooking time to 2 hours on Low settings.
3. Mix well and serve.

**Nutrition Info:**
- Info Per Serving: Calories: 78, Total Fat: 3g, Fiber: 2g, Total Carbs: 9g, Protein: 2g

# Glazed Sausages

Servings: 24 | Cooking Time: 4 Hours

**Ingredients:**
- 10 ounces jarred red pepper jelly
- 1/3 cup bbq sauce
- ½ cup brown sugar
- 16 ounces pineapple chunks and juice
- 24 ounces cocktail-size sausages
- 1 tablespoons cornstarch
- 2 tablespoons water
- Cooking spray

**Directions:**
1. Grease your Crock Pot with cooking spray, add pepper jelly, bbq sauce, brown sugar, pineapple and sausages, stir, cover and cook on Low for 3 hours.
2. Add cornstarch mixed with the water, whisk everything and cook on High for 1 more hour.
3. Arrange sausages on a platter and serve them as a snack.

**Nutrition Info:**
- Info calories 170, fat 10, fiber 1, carbs 17, protein 4

# Cheesy Corn Dip

Servings: 12 | Cooking Time: 4 Hours

**Ingredients:**
- 3 cups corn
- 8 ounces cream cheese, soft
- 1 and ½ cup cheddar cheese, shredded
- ½ cup salsa Verde
- 2 ounces black olives, pitted and sliced
- 1 teaspoon chives, chopped
- Cooking spray

**Directions:**
1. Grease your Crock Pot with the cooking spray, add corn, cream cheese, cheddar, salsa Verde, olives and chives, stir, cover and cook on Low for 4 hours.
2. Divide into bowls and serve as a snack.

**Nutrition Info:**
- Info calories 223, fat 4, fiber 7, carbs 17, protein 5

# Chickpea Hummus

Servings: 10 | Cooking Time: 8 Hrs

**Ingredients:**
- 1 cup chickpeas, dried
- 2 tbsp olive oil
- 3 cup of water
- A pinch of salt and black pepper
- 1 garlic clove, minced
- 1 tbsp lemon juice

**Directions:**
1. Add chickpeas, salt, water, and black pepper to the Crock Pot.
2. Put the cooker's lid on and set the cooking time to 8 hours on Low settings.
3. Drain and transfer the chickpeas to a blender jug.
4. Add salt, black pepper, lemon juice, garlic, and olive oil.
5. Blend the chickpeas dip until smooth.
6. Serve.

**Nutrition Info:**
- Info Per Serving: Calories: 211, Total Fat: 6g, Fiber: 7g, Total Carbs: 8g, Protein: 4g

# Artichoke Dip

Servings: 2 | Cooking Time: 2 Hours

**Ingredients:**
- 2 ounces canned artichoke hearts, drained and chopped
- 2 ounces heavy cream
- 2 tablespoons mayonnaise
- ¼ cup mozzarella, shredded
- 2 green onions, chopped
- ½ teaspoon garam masala
- Cooking spray

**Directions:**
1. Grease your Crock Pot with the cooking spray, and mix the artichokes with the cream, mayo and the other ingredients inside.
2. Stir, cover, cook on Low for 2 hours, divide into bowls and serve as a party dip.

**Nutrition Info:**
- Info calories 100, fat 3, fiber 2, carbs 7, protein 3

# Butter Stuffed Chicken Balls

Servings: 9 | Cooking Time: 3.5 Hours

**Ingredients:**
- 3 oz. butter, cubed
- 1 tbsp mayonnaise
- 1 tsp cayenne pepper
- 1 tsp ground black pepper
- 1 tsp salt
- 1 egg
- 2 oz. white bread
- 4 tbsp milk
- 1 tsp olive oil
- 1 tbsp almond flour
- 1 tsp dried dill
- 14 oz. ground chicken
- ½ tsp olive oil

**Directions:**
1. Whisk mayonnaise with black pepper, dill, chicken, salt, and cayenne pepper in a bowl.
2. Stir in egg, milk, and white bread then mix well.
3. Grease the base of the Crock Pot with cooking oil.
4. Make small meatballs our of this mixture and insert one butter cubes into each ball.
5. Dust the meatballs with almond then place them in the Crock Pot.
6. Put the cooker's lid on and set the cooking time to 3.5 hours on High settings.
7. Serve warm.

**Nutrition Info:**
- Info Per Serving: Calories: 181, Total Fat: 14.1g, Fiber: 1g, Total Carbs: 4.02g, Protein: 10g

# Creamy Mushroom Bites

Servings: 10 | Cooking Time: 5 Hours

**Ingredients:**
- 7 oz. shiitake mushroom, chopped
- 2 eggs
- 1 tbsp cream cheese
- 3 tbsp panko bread crumbs
- 2 tbsp flour
- 1 tsp minced garlic
- 1 tsp salt
- ½ tsp chili flakes
- 1 tsp olive oil
- 1 tsp ground coriander
- ½ tsp nutmeg
- 1 tbsp almond flour
- 1 tsp butter, melted

**Directions:**
1. Toss the mushrooms with salt, chili flakes, olive oil, ground coriander, garlic, and nutmeg in a skillet.
2. Stir cook for 5 minutes approximately on medium heat.
3. Whisk eggs with flour, cream cheese, and bread crumbs in a suitable bowl.
4. Stir in sauteed mushrooms and butter then mix well.
5. Knead this mushroom dough and divide it into golf ball-sized balls.
6. Pour the oil from the skillet in the Crock Pot.
7. Add the mushroom dough balls to the cooker.
8. Put the cooker's lid on and set the cooking time to 3 hours on High settings.
9. Flip the balls and cook for another 2 hours on high heat.
10. Serve.

**Nutrition Info:**
- Info Per Serving: Calories: 65, Total Fat: 3.5g, Fiber: 1g, Total Carbs: 6.01g, Protein: 3g

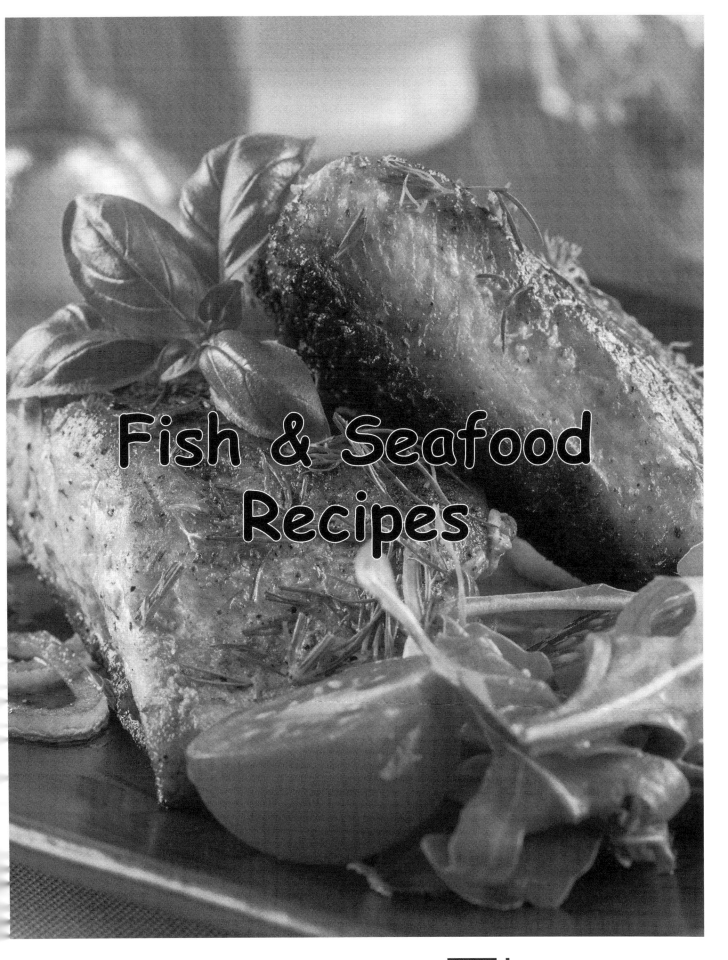

# Fish & Seafood Recipes

# Fish & Seafood Recipes

## Lemony Shrimps In Hoisin Sauce

Servings:4 | Cooking Time: 2 Hours

**Ingredients:**
- 1/3 cup hoisin sauce
- ½ cup lemon juice, freshly squeezed
- 1 ½ pounds shrimps, shelled and deveined
- Salt and pepper to taste
- 2 tablespoon cilantro leaves, chopped

**Directions:**
1. Into the crockpot, place the hoisin sauce, lemon juice, and shrimps.
2. Season with salt and pepper to taste.
3. Mix to incorporate all ingredients.
4. Close the lid and cook on high for 30 minutes or on low for 2 hours.
5. Garnish with cilantro leaves.

**Nutrition Info:**
- Info  Calories per serving: 228; Carbohydrates: 6.3g; Protein: 35.8g; Fat: 3.2g; Sugar: 0g; Sodium: 482mg; Fiber: 4.8g

## Paprika Cod

Servings: 2 | Cooking Time: 3 Hours

**Ingredients:**
- 1 tablespoon olive oil
- 1 pound cod fillets, boneless
- 1 teaspoon sweet paprika
- ¼ cup chicken stock
- ¼ cup white wine
- 2 scallions, chopped
- ½ teaspoon rosemary, dried
- A pinch of salt and black pepper

**Directions:**
1. In your Crock Pot, mix the cod with the paprika, oil and the other ingredients, toss gently, put the lid on and cook on High for 3 hours.
2. Divide everything between plates and serve.

**Nutrition Info:**
- Info calories 211, fat 8, fiber 4, carbs 8, protein 8

## Caribbean Seasoning Fish Balls

Servings:4 | Cooking Time: 3 Hours

**Ingredients:**
- 1 teaspoon Caribbean seasonings
- ½ teaspoon dried thyme
- 12 oz salmon fillet, chopped
- 1 egg, beaten
- 1 teaspoon sunflower oil
- ¼ cup of water

**Directions:**
1. Mix Caribbean seasonings with dried thyme.
2. Then add chopped salmon and carefully mix. Add egg.
3. Pour sunflower oil in the Crock Pot. Add water.
4. Make the fish balls with the help of the spoon and put them in the Crock Pot.
5. Cook the fish balls on High for 3 hours.

**Nutrition Info:**
- InfoPer Serving: 145 calories, 17.9g protein, 1.7g carbohydrates, 0.1g fat, 0.1g fiber, 78mg cholesterol, 161mg sodium, 343mg potassium

# Simple Crockpot Steamed Crab

Servings:2 | Cooking Time: 3 Hours

**Ingredients:**
- 2 pounds medium-sized crabs, cleaned
- Juice from 1 lemon, freshly squeezed
- ¼ cup water
- 3 tablespoons butter
- 4 cloves of garlic, minced
- 2 onions, chopped
- 2 bay leaves
- Salt and pepper to taste

**Directions:**
1. Place all ingredients in the CrockPot.
2. Give a good stir.
3. Close the lid and cook on high for 2 hours or on low for 3 hours.

**Nutrition Info:**
- Info Calories per serving: 392; Carbohydrates: 2.1g; Protein: 38.2g; Fat: 27.5g; Sugar: 0g; Sodium: 819mg; Fiber: 1.6g

# Curry Clams

Servings:4 | Cooking Time: 1.5 Hour

**Ingredients:**
- 1-pound clams
- 1 teaspoon curry paste
- ¼ cup of coconut milk
- 1 cup of water

**Directions:**
1. Mix coconut milk with curry paste and water and pour it in the Crock Pot.
2. Add clams and close the lid.
3. Cook the meal on High for 1.5 hours or until the clams are opened.

**Nutrition Info:**
- InfoPer Serving: 97 calories, 1.1g protein, 13.6g carbohydrates, 4.5g fat, 0.8g fiber, 0mg cholesterol, 415mg sodium, 141mg potassium.

# Pangasius Fish Balls

Servings:4 | Cooking Time: 2.5 Hours

**Ingredients:**
- 10 oz pangasius fillet, minced
- 3 tablespoons breadcrumbs
- 1 teaspoon minced garlic
- ½ teaspoon salt
- 1 tablespoon flour
- 1 tablespoon coconut oil
- ½ cup of water

**Directions:**
1. In the mixing bowl mix fish fillet with minced garlic, bread crumbs, salt, and flour.
2. Make the fish balls.
3. Then heat the coconut oil in the skillet well.
4. Add the fish balls and roast them on high heat for 2 minutes per side.
5. Transfer the fish balls in the Crock Pot.
6. Add water and cook them on High for 2.5 hours.

**Nutrition Info:**
- InfoPer Serving: 107 calories, 10.3g protein, 5.4g carbohydrates, 5.6g fat, 0.3g fiber, 13mg cholesterol, 491mg sodium, 15mg potassium

# Shrimp And Peas Soup

Servings: 4 | Cooking Time: 1 Hour

**Ingredients:**
- 4 scallions, chopped
- 1 tablespoon olive oil
- 1 small ginger root, grated
- 8 cups chicken stock
- ¼ cup soy sauce
- 5 ounces canned bamboo shoots, sliced
- Black pepper to the taste
- ¼ teaspoon fish sauce
- 1 pound shrimp, peeled and deveined
- ½ pound snow peas
- 1 tablespoon sesame oil
- ½ tablespoon chili oil

**Directions:**
1. In your Crock Pot, mix olive oil with scallions, ginger, stock, soy sauce, bamboo, black pepper, fish sauce, shrimp, peas, sesame oil and chili oil, cover and cook on High for 1 hour.
2. Stir soup, ladle into bowls and serve.

**Nutrition Info:**
- Info calories 240, fat 3, fiber 2, carbs 12, protein 14

# Sage Shrimps

Servings:4 | Cooking Time: 1 Hour

**Ingredients:**
- 1-pound shrimps, peeled
- 1 teaspoon dried sage
- 1 teaspoon minced garlic
- 1 teaspoon white pepper
- 1 cup tomatoes chopped
- ½ cup of water

**Directions:**
1. Put all ingredients in the Crock Pot and close the lid.
2. Cook the shrimps on High for 1 hour.

**Nutrition Info:**
- InfoPer Serving: 146 calories, 26.4g protein, 4.1g carbohydrates, 2.1g fat, 0.8g fiber, 239mg cholesterol, 280mg sodium, 310mg potassium.

# Coconut Catfish

Servings:3 | Cooking Time: 2.5 Hours

**Ingredients:**
- 3 catfish fillets
- 1 teaspoon coconut shred
- ½ cup of coconut milk
- 1 teaspoon sesame seeds
- 2 tablespoons fish sauce
- 1 cup of water
- 2 tablespoons soy sauce

**Directions:**
1. Pour water in the Crock Pot.
2. Add soy sauce, fish sauce, sesame seeds, and coconut milk.
3. Then add coconut shred and catfish fillets.
4. Cook the fish on high for 2.5 hours.

**Nutrition Info:**
- InfoPer Serving: 329 calories, 27.3g protein, 3.9g carbohydrates, 22.7g fat, 1.2g fiber, 75mg cholesterol, 1621mg sodium, 682mg potassium.

# Dill Cod Sticks

Servings:4 | Cooking Time: 1.5 Hours

**Ingredients:**
- 4 teaspoons breadcrumbs
- 1 egg, beaten
- 1 tablespoon cream cheese
- ½ teaspoon salt
- 1 teaspoon avocado oil
- ¼ cup of water
- 2 cod fillets

**Directions:**
1. Slice the cod and sprinkle it with salt.
2. Then dip the fish in the egg and coat in the breadcrumbs.
3. Heat the avocado oil in the skillet well.
4. Add the fish sticks and roast them for 1 minute per side.
5. Transfer the fish sticks in the Crock Pot.
6. Add all remaining ingredients and close the lid.
7. Cook the cod sticks on High for 1.5 hours.

**Nutrition Info:**
- InfoPer Serving: 80 calories, 11.9g protein, 1.8g carbohydrates, 2.7g fat, 0.2g fiber, 71mg cholesterol, 365mg sodium, 26mg potassium

# Spicy Tuna

Servings: 2 | Cooking Time: 2 Hours

**Ingredients:**
- 1 pound tuna fillets, boneless and cubed
- ½ teaspoon red pepper flakes, crushed
- ¼ teaspoon cayenne pepper
- ½ cup chicken stock
- ½ teaspoon chili powder
- 1 tablespoon olive oil
- A pinch of salt and black pepper
- 1 tablespoon chives, chopped

**Directions:**
1. In your Crock Pot, mix the tuna with the pepper flakes, cayenne and the other ingredients, toss, put the lid on and cook on High for 2 hours.
2. Divide the tuna mix between plates and serve.

**Nutrition Info:**
- Info calories 193, fat 7, fiber 3, carbs 6, protein 6

# Stuffed Squid

Servings: 4 | Cooking Time: 3 Hours

**Ingredients:**
- 4 squid
- 1 cup sticky rice
- 14 ounces dashi stock
- 2 tablespoons sake
- 4 tablespoons soy sauce
- 1 tablespoon mirin
- 2 tablespoons sugar

**Directions:**
1. Chop tentacles from 1 squid, mix with the rice, stuff each squid with this mix and seal ends with toothpicks.
2. Place squid in your Crock Pot, add stock, soy sauce, sake, sugar and mirin, stir, cover and cook on High for 3 hours.
3. Divide between plates and serve.

**Nutrition Info:**
- Info calories 230, fat 4, fiber 4, carbs 7, protein 11

## Spicy Basil Shrimp

Servings:4 | Cooking Time: 2 Hours

**Ingredients:**
- 1-pound raw shrimp, shelled and deveined
- Salt and pepper to taste
- 1 tablespoon butter
- ¼ cup packed fresh basil leaves
- ¼ teaspoon cayenne pepper

**Directions:**
1. Add all ingredients in the crockpot.
2. Give a stir.
3. Close the lid and cook on high for 30 minutes or on low for 2 hours.

**Nutrition Info:**
- Info Calories per serving: 144; Carbohydrates: 1.4g; Protein: 23.4g; Fat: 6.2g; Sugar: 0g; Sodium: 126mg; Fiber:0.5 g

## Coriander Cod Balls

Servings:3 | Cooking Time: 2 Hours

**Ingredients:**
- ½ teaspoon minced garlic
- 8 oz cod fillet, grinded
- 1 teaspoon dried cilantro
- 2 tablespoons cornflour
- 1 teaspoon avocado oil
- ¼ cup of water

**Directions:**
1. Mix minced garlic with grinded cod, dried cilantro, and cornflour.
2. Make the small balls.
3. After this, heat the avocado oil in the skillet well.
4. Add the fish balls and roast them on high heat for 2 minutes per side.
5. Transfer the fish balls in the Crock Pot.
6. Add water and cook them on High for 2 hours.

**Nutrition Info:**
- InfoPer Serving: 83 calories, 14.4g protein, 4g carbohydrates, 1.1g fat, 0.4g fiber, 39mg cholesterol, 50mg sodium, 23mg potassium

# Shrimp And Mushrooms

Servings: 2 | Cooking Time: 1 Hour

**Ingredients:**
- 1 pound shrimp, peeled and deveined
- 1 cup white mushrooms, halved
- 1 tablespoon avocado oil
- ½ tablespoon tomato paste
- 4 scallions, minced
- ½ cup chicken stock
- Juice of 1 lime
- Salt and black pepper to the taste
- 1 tablespoon chives, minced

**Directions:**
1. In your Crock Pot, mix the shrimp with the mushrooms, oil and the other ingredients, toss, put the lid on and cook on High for 1 hour.
2. Divide the mix into bowls and serve.

**Nutrition Info:**
- Info calories 200, fat 12, fiber 2, carbs 6, protein 9

# Chili Shrimp And Zucchinis

Servings: 4 | Cooking Time: 1 Hour

**Ingredients:**
- 1 pound shrimp, peeled and deveined
- 1 zucchini, cubed
- 2 scallions, minced
- 1 cup tomato passata
- 2 green chilies, chopped
- A pinch of salt and black pepper
- 1 tablespoon chives, chopped

**Directions:**
1. In your Crock Pot, mix the shrimp with the zucchini and the other ingredients, toss, put the lid on and cook on High for 1 hour.
2. Divide the shrimp mix into bowls and serve.

**Nutrition Info:**
- Info calories 210, fat 8, fiber 3, carbs 6, protein 14

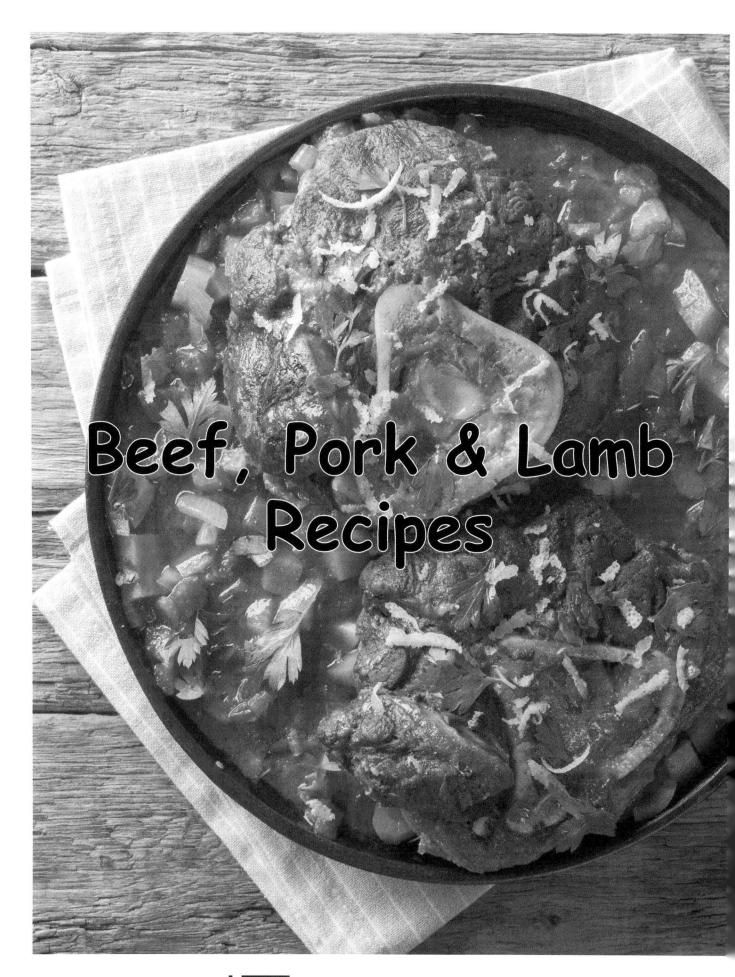

Beef, Pork & Lamb
Recipes

# Beef, Pork & Lamb Recipes

## Lemon Lamb

Servings: 2 | Cooking Time: 7 Hours

**Ingredients:**
- 1 pound lamb stew meat, cubed
- 1 red onion, sliced
- ½ cup tomato sauce
- 1 tablespoon balsamic vinegar
- 1 tablespoon lemon juice
- 1 tablespoon lemon zest, grated
- 1 teaspoon olive oil
- 3 garlic cloves, chopped
- A pinch of salt and black pepper
- 1 tablespoon chives, chopped

**Directions:**
1. In your Crock Pot, mix the lamb with the onion, tomato sauce and the other ingredients, toss, put the lid on and cook on Low for 7 hours.
2. Divide the mix between plates and serve right away.

**Nutrition Info:**
- Info calories 264, fat 8, fiber 3, carbs 6, protein 17

## Carrot And Pork Cubes

Servings:2 | Cooking Time: 4 Hours

**Ingredients:**
- 8 oz pork tenderloin, cubed
- 1 cup carrot, cubed
- 1 tablespoon tomato paste
- 1 tablespoon avocado oil
- 1 teaspoon salt
- 1 teaspoon white pepper

**Directions:**
1. Pour the avocado oil in the skillet and preheat it well.
2. Then put the pork tenderloins in the hot oil and roast on high heat for 3 minutes per side.
3. Transfer the roasted meat in the Crock Pot and add all remaining ingredients.
4. Close the lid and cook the pork on high for 4 hours.

**Nutrition Info:**
- InfoPer Serving: 203 calories, 30.7g protein, 8g carbohydrates, 4.9g fat, 2.3g fiber, 83mg cholesterol, 1274mg sodium, 770mg potassium

## Schweinshaxe

Servings:4 | Cooking Time: 10 Hours

**Ingredients:**
- 1 tablespoon juniper berries
- ½ cup beer
- 1-pound pork knuckle
- ½ teaspoon sugar
- 1 lemon, halved
- 2 cups of water
- 1 tablespoon sunflower oil

**Directions:**
1. Put all ingredients in the Crock Pot and close the lid.
2. Cook the meal on Low for 10 hours.

**Nutrition Info:**
- InfoPer Serving: 311 calories, 29.1g protein, 2.9g carbohydrates, 18.9g fat, 0.4g fiber, 102mg cholesterol, 90mg sodium, 422mg potassium

# Pork Ribs In Soy Sauce

Servings:5 | Cooking Time: 5 Hours

**Ingredients:**
- 1-pound pork ribs
- ½ cup of soy sauce
- ½ cup of water
- 1 onion, sliced
- 1 garlic clove, sliced
- 1 teaspoon sesame seeds
- ½ teaspoon sugar
- ½ teaspoon chili powder

**Directions:**
1. Put all ingredients in the Crock Pot and carefully stir them with the help of the spatula.
2. After this, close the lid and cook the pork ribs on high for 5 hours.
3. When the pork ribs are cooked, transfer them in the bowls and top with soy sauce liquid.

**Nutrition Info:**
- InfoPer Serving: 277 calories, 26.1g protein, 4.9g carbohydrates, 16.4g fat, 0.8g fiber, 93mg cholesterol, 1494mg sodium, 359mg potassium

# Lamb Shoulder

Servings: 6 | Cooking Time: 8 Hours And 10 Minutes

**Ingredients:**
- 3 pounds lamb shoulder, boneless
- 3 onions, roughly chopped
- 1 tablespoon olive oil
- 1 tablespoon oregano, chopped
- 6 garlic cloves, minced
- 1 tablespoon lemon zest, grated
- Salt and black pepper to the taste
- ½ teaspoon allspice
- 1 and ½ cups veggie stock
- 14 ounces canned artichoke hearts, chopped
- ¼ cup tomato paste
- 2 tablespoons parsley, chopped

**Directions:**
1. Heat up a pan with the oil over medium-high heat, add lamb, brown for 5 minutes on each side, transfer to your Crock Pot, add onion, lemon zest, garlic, a pinch of salt, pepper, oregano, allspice, stock and tomato paste, cover and cook on Low for 7 hours and 45 minutes.
2. Add artichokes and parsley, stir gently, cover, cook on Low for 15 more minutes, divide into bowls and serve hot.

**Nutrition Info:**
- Info calories 370, fat 4, fiber 5, carbs 12, protein 16

# Bacon Beef Strips

Servings:4 | Cooking Time: 5 Hours

**Ingredients:**
- 1-pound beef tenderloin, cut into strips
- 4 oz bacon, sliced
- 1 teaspoon salt
- ½ teaspoon ground black pepper
- ½ cup of water

**Directions:**
1. Mix beef with salt and ground black pepper.
2. Then wrap every beef strip with sliced bacon and arrange it in the Crock Pot.
3. Add water and close the lid.
4. Cook the meal on High for 5 hours.

**Nutrition Info:**
- InfoPer Serving: 258 calories,28.9g protein, 0.4g carbohydrates, 14.8g fat, 0.1g fiber, 90mg cholesterol, 869mg sodium, 379mg potassium.

# Roast And Pepperoncinis

Servings: 4 | Cooking Time: 8 Hours

**Ingredients:**
- 5 pounds beef chuck roast
- 1 tablespoon soy sauce
- 10 pepperoncinis
- 1 cup beef stock
- 2 tablespoons butter, melted

**Directions:**
1. In your Crock Pot, mix beef roast with soy sauce, pepperoncinis, stock and butter, toss well, cover and cook on Low for 8 hours.
2. Transfer roast to a cutting board, shred using2 forks, return to Crock Pot, toss, divide between plates and serve.

**Nutrition Info:**
- Info calories 362, fat 4, fiber 8, carbs 17, protein 17

# Simple Roast Beef

Servings:4 | Cooking Time:  12 Hours

**Ingredients:**
- 2 pounds rump roast
- 1 cup onion, chopped
- 3 tablespoons butter
- Salt and pepper to taste
- ¼ cup water

**Directions:**
1. Place all ingredients in the crockpot.
2. Give a good stir.
3. Close the lid and cook on low for 12 hours or on high for 10 hours.
4. Once cooked, shred the pot roast using two forks.
5. Return to the crockpot and continue cooking on high for 1 hour.

**Nutrition Info:**
- Info  Calories per serving: 523; Carbohydrates:1.8g; Protein: 43.6g; Fat: 32.6g; Sugar: 0g; Sodium: 734mg; Fiber:1.2 g

# Blanked Hot Dogs

Servings:4 | Cooking Time: 4 Hours

**Ingredients:**
- 4 mini (cocktail) pork sausages
- 1 teaspoon cumin seeds
- 1 tablespoon olive oil
- 1 egg, beaten
- 4 oz puff pastry

**Directions:**
1. Roll up the puff pastry and cut into strips.
2. Put the pork sausages on every strip.
3. Roll the puff pastry and brush with egg.
4. Then top the blanked hot dogs with cumin seeds.
5. Brush the Crock Pot with olive oil from inside.
6. Add the blanked hot dogs and close the lid.
7. Cook them on high for 4 hours.

**Nutrition Info:**
- InfoPer Serving: 225 calories, 4.4g protein, 14.1g carbohydrates, 16.9g fat, 0.6g fiber, 41mg cholesterol, 120mg sodium, 42mg potassium

# Ginger Beef

Servings:2 | Cooking Time: 4.5 Hours

**Ingredients:**
- 10 oz beef brisket, sliced
- 1 teaspoon minced ginger
- 1 teaspoon ground coriander
- 1 tablespoon olive oil
- 1 tablespoon lemon juice
- 1 cup of water

**Directions:**
1. In the bowl mix lemon juice and olive oil.
2. Then mix beef brisket with ground coriander and minced ginger.
3. Sprinkle the meat with oil mixture and transfer in the Crock Pot.
4. Add water and cook the meal on High for 5 hours.

**Nutrition Info:**
- InfoPer Serving: 328 calories, 43.1g protein, 0.8g carbohydrates, 15.9g fat, 0.1g fiber, 127mg cholesterol, 99mg sodium, 595mg potassium.

# Short Ribs With Tapioca Sauce

Servings: 6 | Cooking Time: 10 Hrs.

**Ingredients:**
- 3 lbs. beef short ribs
- 1 fennel bulb, cut into wedges
- 2 yellow onions, cut into wedges
- 1 cup carrot, sliced
- 14 oz. canned tomatoes, chopped
- 1 cup dry red wine
- 2 tbsp tapioca, crushed
- 2 tbsp tomato paste
- 1 tsp rosemary, dried
- Salt and black pepper to the taste
- 4 garlic cloves, minced

**Directions:**
1. Add short ribs, onion, and all other ingredients to the insert of Crock Pot.
2. Put the cooker's lid on and set the cooking time to 10 hours on Low settings.
3. Serve warm.

**Nutrition Info:**
- Info Per Serving: Calories: 432, Total Fat: 14g, Fiber: 6g, Total Carbs: 25g, Protein: 42g

# Lamb Saute

Servings:5 | Cooking Time: 4.5 Hours

**Ingredients:**
- 1 cup tomatoes, chopped
- 1 cup bell pepper, chopped
- 1 chili pepper, chopped
- 1 tablespoon avocado oil
- 12 oz lamb fillet, chopped
- ½ cup cremini mushrooms, sliced
- 1 cup of water

**Directions:**
1. Heat the avocado oil in the skillet well.
2. Add chopped lamb and roast it for 5 minutes. Stir the meat from time to time.
3. After this, transfer the meat in the Crock Pot and add all remaining ingredients.
4. Close the lid and cook the saute on High for 5 hours.

**Nutrition Info:**
- InfoPer Serving: 147 calories, 19.9g protein, 3.7g carbohydrates, 5.5g fat, 0.9g fiber, 61mg cholesterol, 56mg sodium, 402mg potassium.

# Chili Beef Sausages

Servings:5 | Cooking Time: 4 Hours

**Ingredients:**
- 1-pound beef sausages
- 1 tablespoon olive oil
- ¼ cup of water
- 1 teaspoon chili powder

**Directions:**
1. Pour olive oil in the Crock Pot.
2. Then sprinkle the beef sausages with chili powder and put in the Crock Pot.
3. Add water and close the lid.
4. Cook the beef sausages on high for 4 hours.

**Nutrition Info:**
- InfoPer Serving: 385 calories, 12.6g protein, 2.7g carbohydrates, 35.8g fat, 0.2g fiber, 64mg cholesterol, 736mg sodium, 182mg potassium.

# 5-ingredients Chili

Servings:4 | Cooking Time: 5 Hours

**Ingredients:**
- 8 oz ground beef
- ½ cup Cheddar cheese, shredded
- 2 cup tomatoes, chopped
- 1 teaspoon chili seasonings
- ½ cup of water

**Directions:**
1. Mix the ground beef with chili seasonings and transfer in the Crock Pot.
2. Add tomatoes and water.
3. Close the lid and cook the chili on high for 3 hours.
4. After this, open the lid and mix the chili well. Top it with cheddar cheese and close the lid.
5. Cook the chili on low for 2 hours more.

**Nutrition Info:**
- InfoPer Serving: 180 calories, 21.6g protein, 4g carbohydrates, 8.4g fat, 1.1g fiber, 66mg cholesterol, 150mg sodium, 456mg potassium.

# Smothered Pepper Steak

Servings:4 | Cooking Time: 10 Hours

**Ingredients:**
- 1 can diced tomatoes
- 1 package bell peppers
- Salt and pepper to taste
- 1 tablespoon soy sauce
- 4 sirloin patties

**Directions:**
1. Place the diced tomatoes (juices and all) in the crockpot.
2. Add the bell peppers. Season with salt, pepper, and soy sauce.
3. Arrange the sirloin patties on top.
4. Close the lid and cook on low for 10 hours or on high for 7 hours.

**Nutrition Info:**
- Info  Calories per serving: 387; Carbohydrates: 5g; Protein: 24.1g; Fat: 18.5g; Sugar: 0.8g; Sodium: 462mg; Fiber: 2.7g

# Mayo Pork Salad

Servings:4 | Cooking Time: 4 Hours

**Ingredients:**
- 7 oz pork loin
- 1 teaspoon salt
- 1 cup of water
- 1 cup arugula, chopped
- 2 eggs, hard-boiled, peeled, chopped
- 3 tablespoons mayonnaise

**Directions:**
1. Pour water in the Crock Pot.
2. Add pork loin and close the lid.
3. Cook the meat on high for 4 hours.
4. After this, drain water and cut the pork loin into strips.
5. Put the pork strips in the big salad bowl.
6. Add arugula and chopped eggs.
7. Add mayonnaise and carefully mix the salad.

**Nutrition Info:**
- InfoPer Serving: 196 calories, 16.6g protein, 3g carbohydrates, 12.8g fat, 0.1g fiber, 124mg cholesterol, 724mg sodium, 259mg potassium

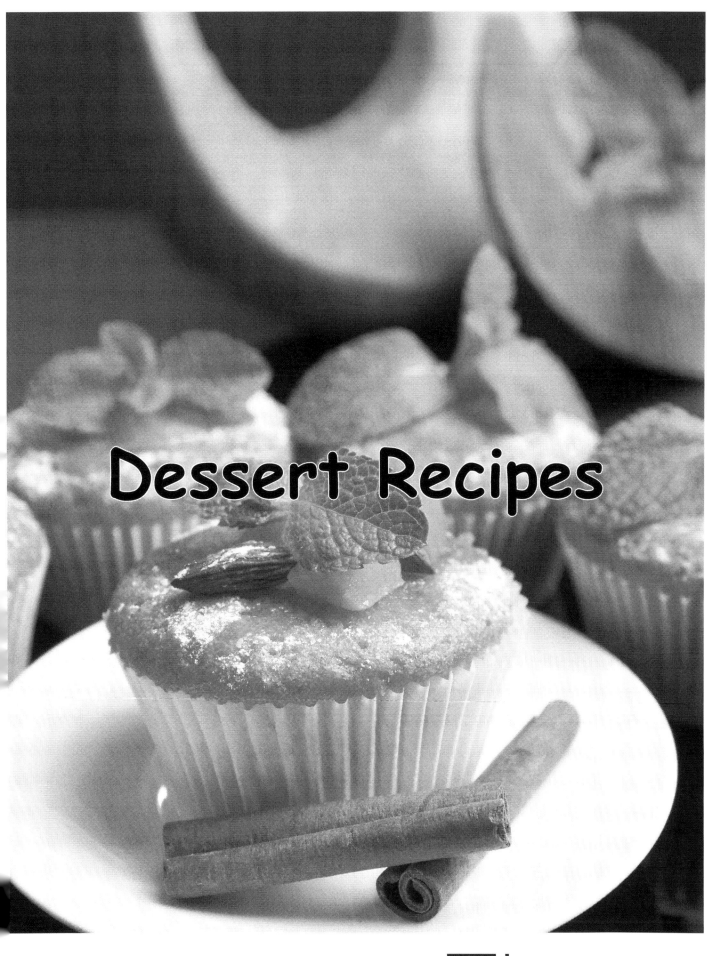

# Dessert Recipes

# Dessert Recipes

## Molten Chocolate Cake

Servings 6

Cooking Time 2 12 Hours

**Ingredients:**
- 4 eggs
- 12 cup butter, melted
- 1 teaspoon vanilla extract
- 1 cup sugar
- 1 cup all-purpose flour
- 14 cup cocoa powder
- 1 teaspoon baking powder
- 14 teaspoon salt

**Directions:**
1. Mix the eggs, butter, vanilla and sugar in a bowl until creamy.
2. Add the flour, cocoa powder and salt and give it just a quick mix, making sure not to over mix the batter.
3. Pour the batter in your crock pot and cook on high settings for 2 hours.
4. The cake is best served warm.

## Orange And Apricot Jam

Servings:4 | Cooking Time: 3 Hours

**Ingredients:**
- 2 oranges, peeled, chopped
- 1 cup apricots, chopped
- 1 tablespoon orange zest, grated
- 4 tablespoons sugar

**Directions:**
1. Put all ingredients in the bowl and blend them until smooth with the help of the immersion blender.
2. Then pour the mixture in the Crock Pot and cook it on High for 3 hours.
3. Transfer the hot jam in the glass cans and close with a lid.
4. Cool the jam well.

**Nutrition Info:**
- InfoPer Serving: 108 calories, 1.4g protein, 27.4g carbohydrates, 0.4g fat, 3.1g fiber, 0mg cholesterol, 1mg sodium, 270mg potassium.

## Cinnamon Apples

Servings: 2 | Cooking Time: 2 Hours

**Ingredients:**
- 2 tablespoons brown sugar
- 1 pound apples, cored and cut into wedges
- 1 tablespoon cinnamon powder
- 2 tablespoons walnuts, chopped
- A pinch of nutmeg, ground
- ½ tablespoon lemon juice
- ¼ cup water
- 2 apples, cored and tops cut off

**Directions:**
1. In your Crock Pot, mix the apples with the sugar, cinnamon and the other ingredients, toss, put the lid on and cook on High for 2 hours.
2. Divide the mix between plates and serve.

**Nutrition Info:**
- Info calories 189, fat 4, fiber 7, carbs 19, protein 2

# Chunky Pumpkin Cake

Servings: 8 | Cooking Time: 5 1/2 Hours

**Ingredients:**

- 3 eggs
- 1/2 cup canola oil
- 2/3 cup white sugar
- 1 cup sour cream
- 1 1/2 cups all-purpose flour
- 1 teaspoon baking powder
- 1/4 teaspoon salt
- 1/2 teaspoon cinnamon powder
- 1/4 teaspoon ground ginger
- 1/4 teaspoon ground cloves
- 2 cups pumpkin cubes

**Directions:**

1. Mix the eggs, sugar and oil in a bowl for 5 minutes until double in volume.
2. Stir in the sour cream then add the flour, baking powder, salt and spices.
3. Pour the batter in your crock pot.
4. Top with pumpkin cubes and cook on low settings for 5 hours.
5. Allow the cake to cool before slicing and serving.

# Spiced Rice Pudding

Servings: 6 | Cooking Time: 4 1/4 Hours

**Ingredients:**

- 1 cup Arborio rice
- 1/2 cup white sugar
- 3 cups whole milk
- 1 cinnamon stick
- 1 star anise
- 2 whole cloves
- 1/2-inch piece of ginger, sliced
- 1/2 teaspoon rose water

**Directions:**

1. Combine all the ingredients in your Crock Pot.
2. Cover the pot and cook on low settings for 4 hours.
3. The pudding can be served both warm and chilled.

# Upside Down Banana Cake

Servings: 8 | Cooking Time: 4 1/2 Hours

**Ingredients:**

- 2 ripe bananas, sliced
- 1/2 cup light brown sugar
- 2 tablespoons brandy
- 1/2 cup butter
- 3/4 cup sugar
- 2 eggs
- 3/4 cup sour cream
- 1 teaspoon vanilla extract
- 1 cup all-purpose flour
- 1/4 cup cornstarch
- 1 teaspoon baking soda
- 1 pinch salt

**Directions:**

1. Spread the brown sugar in your Crock Pot.
2. Arrange the banana slices over the sugar and drizzle with brandy.
3. For the cake, mix the butter and 3/4 cup sugar in a bowl until creamy, at least 3 minutes.
4. Add the eggs, one by one, followed by the sour cream and vanilla.
5. Fold in the flour, cornstarch, baking soda and salt then spoon the batter over the banana slices.
6. Cover the pot and cook on low settings for 4 hours.
7. Allow the cake to cool for 10 minutes then carefully turn it upside down on a platter. You can also slice it and serve it straight from the pot.

# Latte Vanilla Cake

Servings: 7 | Cooking Time: 7 Hrs.

**Ingredients:**
- ½ cup pumpkin puree
- 3 cups flour
- 4 eggs
- 1 cup sugar, brown
- ½ cup of coconut milk
- 4 tbsp olive oil
- 3 tbsp espresso powder
- 2 tbsp maple syrup
- 1 tbsp vanilla extract
- 4 tbsp liquid honey
- ¼ tsp cooking spray

**Directions:**
1. Beat eggs with pumpkin puree, espresso powder, and brown sugar in a bowl.
2. Stir in olive oil, coconut milk, vanilla extract, liquid honey, flour, and maple syrup.
3. Whisk this pumpkin batter using a hand mixer until smooth.
4. Use cooking to grease the insert of your Crock Pot and pour the batter in it.
5. Put the cooker's lid on and set the cooking time to 7 hours on Low settings.
6. Slice and serve when chilled.

**Nutrition Info:**
- Info Per Serving: Calories: 538, Total Fat: 22g, Fiber: 2g, Total Carbs: 71.97g, Protein: 14g

# Spiced Peach Crisp

Servings: 6 | Cooking Time: 3.5 Hrs.

**Ingredients:**
- 1 lb. peaches, pitted and sliced
- ¼ cup of sugar
- 4 tbsp lemon juice
- 1 tsp vanilla extract
- 5 oz oats
- 1 tsp baking soda
- 1 tsp vinegar
- 1/3 cup flour
- 3 tbsp butter
- 1 tsp ground ginger
- ½ tsp pumpkin pie seasoning

**Directions:**
1. Grease the insert of Crock Pot with butter.
2. Place the peach slices in the insert and top them with sugar and lemon juice.
3. Toss oats with vanilla extract, vinegar, baking soda, flour, ground ginger, pumpkin pie seasoning in a bowl.
4. Spread this oats spice mixture on top of the peaches.
5. Put the cooker's lid on and set the cooking time to 1.5 hours on High settings.
6. Remove the lid and stir the cooked mixture well.
7. Cover again and continue cooking for another 2 hours on High settings.
8. Serve.

**Nutrition Info:**
- Info Per Serving: Calories: 212, Total Fat: 7.6g, Fiber: 5g, Total Carbs: 41.26g, Protein: 5g

# Coconut Jam

Servings: 2 | Cooking Time: 3 Hours

**Ingredients:**
- ½ cup coconut flesh, shredded
- 1 cup coconut cream
- ½ cup heavy cream
- 3 tablespoons sugar
- 1 tablespoon lemon juice

**Directions:**
1. In your Crock Pot, mix the coconut cream with the lemon juice and the other ingredients, whisk, put the lid on and cook on Low for 3 hours.
2. Whisk well, divide into bowls and serve cold.

**Nutrition Info:**
- Info calories 50, fat 1, fiber 1, carbs 10, protein 2

# Overnight Plum Pudding

Servings: 8 | Cooking Time: 8 1/4 Hours

**Ingredients:**
- 1 1/2 cups all-purpose flour
- 1/4 cup dark brown sugar
- 1/2 teaspoon baking soda
- 4 tablespoons butter, softened
- 2 eggs
- 1 cup mixed dried fruits, chopped
- 1/2 cup dried plums, chopped
- 1 cup hot water

**Directions:**
1. Mix the dried fruits, plums and hot water in a bowl and allow to soak up for 10 minutes.
2. Combine the flour, brown sugar, baking soda, butter, eggs and the dried fruits plus the water in a large bowl.
3. Mix well with a spoon or spatula then spoon the batter in your crock pot.
4. Cover and cook on low settings for 8 hours.
5. Allow the pudding to cool in the pot before serving.

# Strawberry Cake

Servings: 2 | Cooking Time: 1 Hour

**Ingredients:**
- ¼ cup coconut flour
- ¼ teaspoon baking soda
- 1 tablespoon sugar
- ¼ cup strawberries, chopped
- ½ cup coconut milk
- 1 teaspoon butter, melted
- ½ teaspoon lemon zest, grated
- ¼ teaspoon vanilla extract
- Cooking spray

**Directions:**
1. In a bowl, mix the coconut flour with the baking soda, sugar and the other ingredients except the cooking spray and stir well.
2. Grease your Crock Pot with the cooking spray, line it with parchment paper, pour the cake batter inside, put the lid on and cook on High for 1 hour.
3. Leave the cake to cool down, slice and serve.

**Nutrition Info:**
- Info calories 200, fat 4, fiber 4, carbs 10, protein 4

# Banana Chunk Cake

Servings: 10 | Cooking Time: 3 1/4 Hours

**Ingredients:**
- 1/2 cup butter, softened
- 1/2 cup brown sugar
- 1/4 cup white sugar
- 2 eggs
- 2 tablespoons dark rum
- 1/4 cup milk
- 1 cup all-purpose flour
- 1 teaspoon baking powder
- 1/2 teaspoon salt
- 2 ripe bananas, sliced
- 1/2 cup dark chocolate chips

**Directions:**
1. Mix the butter and sugars in a bowl for a few minutes until creamy.
2. Add the eggs, rum and milk and give it a quick mix.
3. Fold in the flour, salt and baking powder then add the banana and chocolate chips.
4. Pour the batter in your greased Crock Pot and cook on high settings for 3 hours.
5. Serve the cake chilled.

# Orange Curd

Servings:6 | Cooking Time: 7 Hours

**Ingredients:**
- 2 cups orange juice
- 1 tablespoon orange zest, grated
- 4 egg yolks
- 1 cup of sugar
- 1 tablespoon cornflour
- 1 teaspoon vanilla extract

**Directions:**
1. Whisk the egg yolks with sugar until you get a lemon color mixture.
2. Then add orange juice, vanilla extract, cornflour, and orange zest. Whisk the mixture until smooth.
3. Pour the liquid in the Crock Pot and close the lid.
4. Cook the curd on low for 7 hours. Stir the curd every 1 hour.

**Nutrition Info:**
- InfoPer Serving: 206 calories, 2.5g protein, 43.6g carbohydrates, 3.2g fat, 0.4g fiber, 140mg cholesterol, 6mg sodium, 185mg potassium.

# Poppy Cream Pie

Servings: 6 | Cooking Time: 6 Hrs.

**Ingredients:**
- 5 tbsp poppy seeds
- 3 egg, whisked
- 1 cup cream cheese
- 1 cup flour
- 1 tsp baking soda
- 1 cup of sugar
- 1 tbsp orange juice
- 1 tsp butter
- 3 tbsp heavy cream
- 1 pinch salt

**Directions:**
1. Whisk cream cheese with eggs, baking soda, and sugar in a mixer.
2. Stir in butter, heavy cream, salt, and orange juice, then mix until smooth.
3. Fold in poppy seeds and mix gently.
4. Layer the insert of Crock Pot with a parchment sheet.
5. Spread the poppy seeds batter in the insert of the cooker.
6. Put the cooker's lid on and set the cooking time to 6 hours on Low settings.
7. Slice and serve when chilled.

**Nutrition Info:**
- Info Per Serving: Calories: 395, Total Fat: 22.9g, Fiber: 2g, Total Carbs: 37.01g, Protein: 11g

# Sweet Cookies

Servings: 10 | Cooking Time: 2 Hours And 30 Minutes

**Ingredients:**
- 1 egg white
- ¼ cup vegetable oil
- 1 cup sugar
- ½ teaspoon vanilla extract
- 1 teaspoon baking powder
- 1 and ½ cups almond meal
- ½ cup dark chocolate chips

**Directions:**
1. In a bowl, mix coconut oil with sugar, vanilla extract and egg white and beat well using your mixer.
2. Add baking powder and almond meal and stir well.
3. Fold in chocolate chips and stir gently.
4. Line your Crock Pot with parchment paper and grease it.
5. Transfer cookie mix to your Crock Pot, press it on the bottom, cover and cook on low for 2 hours and 30 minutes.
6. Take cookie sheet out of the Crock Pot, cut in 10 bars and serve.

**Nutrition Info:**
- Info calories 220, fat 2, fiber 1, carbs 3, protein 6

# Pudding Cake

Servings: 8 | Cooking Time: 2 Hours And 30 Minutes

**Ingredients:**
- 1 and ½ cup sugar
- 1 cup flour
- ¼ cup cocoa powder+ 2 tablespoons
- ½ cup chocolate almond milk
- 2 teaspoons baking powder
- 2 tablespoons vegetable oil
- 1 teaspoon vanilla extract
- 1 and ½ cups hot water
- Cooking spray

**Directions:**
1. In a bowl, mix flour with 2 tablespoons cocoa, baking powder, milk, oil and vanilla extract, whisk well and spread on the bottom of the Crock Pot, greased with cooking spray.
2. In another bowl, mix sugar with the rest of the cocoa and the water, whisk well, spread over the batter in the Crock Pot, cover, cook your cake on High for 2 hours and 30 minutes.
3. Leave the cake to cool down, slice and serve.

**Nutrition Info:**
- Info calories 250, fat 4, fiber 3, carbs 40, protein 4

## BASIC KITCHEN CONVERSIONS & EQUIVALENTS

### DRY MEASUREMENTS CONVERSION CHART

3 TEASPOONS = 1 TABLESPOON = 1/16 CUP

6 TEASPOONS = 2 TABLESPOONS = 1/8 CUP

12 TEASPOONS = 4 TABLESPOONS = 1/4 CUP

24 TEASPOONS = 8 TABLESPOONS = 1/2 CUP

36 TEASPOONS = 12 TABLESPOONS = 3/4 CUP

48 TEASPOONS = 16 TABLESPOONS = 1 CUP

## METRIC TO US COOKING CONVERSIONS

### OVEN TEMPERATURES

120 °C = 250 °F

160 °C = 320 °F

180° C = 350 °F

205 °C = 400 °F

220 °C = 425 °F

### LIQUID MEASUREMENTS CONVERSION CHART

8 FLUID OUNCES = 1 CUP = 1/2 PINT = 1/4 QUART

16 FLUID OUNCES = 2 CUPS = 1 PINT = 1/2 QUART

32 FLUID OUNCES = 4 CUPS = 2 PINTS = 1 QUART

 = 1/4 GALLON

128 FLUID OUNCES = 16 CUPS = 8 PINTS = 4 QUARTS  = 1 GALLON

### BAKING IN GRAMS

1 CUP FLOUR = 140 GRAMS

1 CUP SUGAR = 150 GRAMS

1 CUP POWDERED SUGAR = 160 GRAMS

1 CUP HEAVY CREAM = 235 GRAMS

### VOLUME

1 MILLILITER = 1/5 TEASPOON

5 ML = 1 TEASPOON

15 ML = 1 TABLESPOON

240 ML = 1 CUP OR 8 FLUID OUNCES

1 LITER = 34 FL. OUNCES

### WEIGHT

1 GRAM = .035 OUNCES

100 GRAMS = 3.5 OUNCES

500 GRAMS = 1.1 POUNDS

1 KILOGRAM = 35 OUNCES

## US TO METRIC COOKING CONVERSIONS

1/5 TSP = 1 ML

1 TSP = 5 ML

1 TBSP = 15 ML

1 FL OUNCE = 30 ML

1 CUP = 237 ML

1 PINT (2 CUPS) = 473 ML

1 QUART (4 CUPS) = .95 LITER

1 GALLON (16 CUPS) = 3.8 LITERS

1 OZ = 28 GRAMS

1 POUND = 454 GRAMS

## BUTTER

1 CUP BUTTER = 2 STICKS = 8 OUNCES = 230 GRAMS = 8 TABLESPOONS

## WHAT DOES 1 CUP EQUAL

1 CUP = 8 FLUID OUNCES

1 CUP = 16 TABLESPOONS

1 CUP = 48 TEASPOONS

1 CUP = 1/2 PINT

1 CUP = 1/4 QUART

1 CUP = 1/16 GALLON

1 CUP = 240 ML

## BAKING PAN CONVERSIONS

1 CUP ALL-PURPOSE FLOUR = 4.5 OZ

1 CUP ROLLED OATS = 3 OZ 1 LARGE EGG = 1.7 OZ

1 CUP BUTTER = 8 OZ 1 CUP MILK = 8 OZ

1 CUP HEAVY CREAM = 8.4 OZ

1 CUP GRANULATED SUGAR = 7.1 OZ

1 CUP PACKED BROWN SUGAR = 7.75 OZ

1 CUP VEGETABLE OIL = 7.7 OZ

1 CUP UNSIFTED POWDERED SUGAR = 4.4 OZ

## BAKING PAN CONVERSIONS

9-INCH ROUND CAKE PAN = 12 CUPS

10-INCH TUBE PAN =16 CUPS

11-INCH BUNDT PAN = 12 CUPS

9-INCH SPRINGFORM PAN = 10 CUPS

9 X 5 INCH LOAF PAN = 8 CUPS

9-INCH SQUARE PAN = 8 CUPS

# Appendix B : Recipes Index

# D

# Q

# R

# S

Made in the USA
Monee, IL
07 October 2023

44137392R00055